REMEMBERING WHAT MATTERS

STORIES FROM AN AMAZING PLACE

REVEAL THE UNEXPECTED

LESSONS

OF DEMENTIA

✦

SUZY LAFORGE

Proceeds from the sale of this book
benefit the cognitive and emotional well-being
of the participants at Amazing Place.

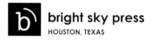

2365 Rice Blvd., Suite 202
Houston, Texas 77005

ISBN: 978-1-942945-41-3

10   9   8   7   6   5   4   3   2   1

Library of Congress Cataloging-in-Publication Data on file with publisher.

Editorial Direction, Lucy Herring Chambers
Managing Editor, Lauren Adams Gow
Designer, Sharon Tooley
Layout, Marla Y. Garcia
Photography, Cindy Crofford
Dove Cover Art by Amazing Place Participant, Huguette Vigeant

Printed in Korea through Four Colour Print Group

DEDICATION

*This book is dedicated to the
countless individuals and organizations
that have made Amazing Place,
the unique day center for adults
with mild to moderate dementia in
Houston, Texas, a reality.
They include the:*

*Visionary Founders
Guiding Board
Sponsoring Churches
Generous Donors
Faithful Volunteers
Caring Staff
Resilient Caregivers
and, Courageous Participants,
who all make
these stories possible.*

ABOUT THIS AMAZING PLACE

It was 1994. It's hard to believe just over twenty years ago, the words "dementia" and "Alzheimer's" were rarely uttered. It was before the news and statistics about how the incidence of this disease is exploding became widespread. It was before one of the top worries of all baby boomers became *Is this a "senior moment" or am I losing my memory for good?* It was before support services became available for families who were dealing, often in silence, with this disease for which there still is no effective prevention, treatment or cure.

A visionary Houston pastor, Rev. Dean Robinson at St. Luke's United Methodist Church, recognized the needs of the growing number of families in his congregation who were facing the challenges of a loved one's memory loss. He realized how these men and women, who could no longer work, needed a safe place for social, physical and mental stimulation. In addition, he saw firsthand how the caregiving families needed emotional support and well-deserved time off.

Two years later, with the help of several founding committee members, Rev. Robinson founded The Seniors Place Adult Day Center. There were three "participants," as the individuals with dementia who attend were and are still called, and three staff members in two converted Sunday School classrooms. Today, that same organization, now called Amazing Place, serves over 3,000 individuals each year through its dementia day program, caregiver support programs and community education.

The mission of enriching lives by providing fellowship, memory care and wellness to those with mild to moderate dementia and support to their families and the community continues today.

DAY PROGRAM

Each week, Monday through Friday, sixty or so participants, ranging in age from forty-nine to ninety-nine and diagnosed with various types of mild to moderate dementia, arrive to attend a stimulating day program in a beautiful modern building that was designed specifically for them. The curriculum allows individuals to choose from a diverse array of activities, depending on their interests and strengths. The backbone of the program is to add structure, socialization and mental, physical, spiritual and creative stimulation to their lives, all of which research has determined are essential for those with dementia.

Classes include:

Cognitive—book clubs, current events and history discussions, word games

Exercise—Tai Chi, Pilates, strength training, cycling, balance

Creative—painting, music, creative writing

Spiritual—daily bible study, daily devotionals, worship services

Recreation—bridge, dominoes, shuffleboard, basketball, putting green

Culture—outings to museums, arts performances

Intergenerational Collaborations—student volunteers and visits
with students from elementary school to college

In addition to the invigorating curriculum, participants are served a three course "Brain Healthy" lunch and snacks each day, following the strict guidelines of the Memory Preservation Nutrition® Program. A full-time registered nurse monitors each participant's medical and medication needs.

CAREGIVER SUPPORT

The day program not only benefits the individuals with dementia, but also provides much-needed respite for their caregivers. Amazing Place also offers monthly support groups, courses on caregiving and stress relief and individual and family counseling from our licensed clinical social worker.

COMMUNITY OUTREACH

Amazing Place has been at the forefront of educating professionals and the community about brain health and dementia. In addition to functioning as a clinical training site to nursing and medical students, we provide educational programming to other professionals needing counsel about working with adults with mild to moderate dementia. Finally, through our "Brain Health Matters" Speakers Bureau, we offer presentations to the community about brain-healthy living and the disease, while working to destigmatize the word "dementia" and encourage early intervention.

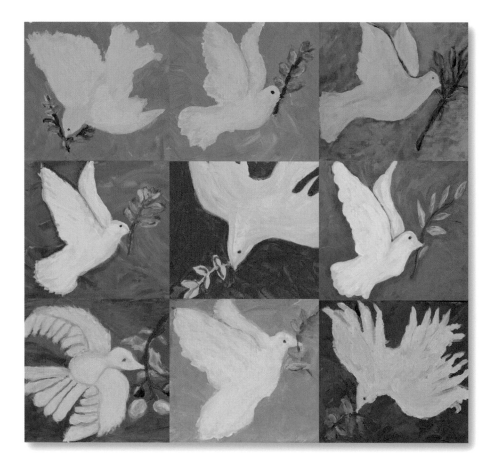

ABOUT THE DOVES

The dove, recreated by our participant artists in the paintings throughout this book,
was selected for our logo as a symbol of a safe place to land and a place of hope—
for both individuals diagnosed with dementia and their families.

TABLE OF CONTENTS

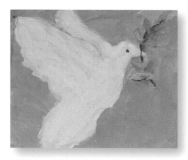 Chances are you or someone you know has faced dementia in a friend or family member. The more than five million Americans with dementia—whether it is Alzheimer's disease, vascular dementia, frontotemporal disease (FTD) or one of a number of other types—translates to over fifteen million* caregivers and loved ones affected by the disease. The emotional, physical and financial toll for caregivers and families can be overwhelming, especially because this disease is the only one of the ten most frequently occurring diseases in the US* with no effective prevention, treatment or cure. And for those who are aware of their diminishing brain, there is nothing more terrifying.

I am one of those millions who have been touched by dementia in a family member— in fact, in both my parents. Like many others, I experienced the grief of watching the mind and behavior of someone I love change before my eyes. But, what also struck me was how much fear, shame and stigma were connected to the mention of dementia. It reminded me of the way I understood cancer had been perceived in the 1960s, and how AIDS was seen in the 1980s. In an extraordinary statistic, I learned that most people living with Alzheimer's disease are not even aware of their diagnosis, although one in three seniors will die with Alzheimer's or another type of dementia.

I saw how easy, and how prevalent, it was for someone to hide, deny or compensate for their symptoms. I witnessed family members who were often reluctant to admit there was a serious problem with a loved one. And, I observed, firsthand, how others were uncomfortable and unsure of how to react to someone who couldn't hold a conversation or would repeat the same thing over and over. To many, it seemed a diagnosis with dementia was "the end."

When my father, who suffered from FTD, was missing and eventually found after wandering down a busy Houston street, we found Amazing Place, in desperation. Amazing Place became not only a safe haven for him, but also a place

*Alzheimer's Association. 2016 Alzheimer's Disease Fact and Figures. *www.alz.org*

that offered him fellowship, stimulation and oversight of his medical care. Literally a life-saver for my father, it also benefitted my mother, who was overwhelmed with the pressures of being a caregiver. I, in turn, as the "front-line family member" felt obvious relief that he would be safe.

The first time I picked him up from what was then called The Seniors Place, I felt an apprehension similar to the feeling of picking my child up from the first day of preschool. Here was a seventy-year-old, formerly brilliant chemical engineer and marketing executive who was going to a place to be "supervised." However, when I picked him up that day, he proudly held some artwork in his hand he had done for my mother and said he had a great day. It still took me awhile to break out of my denial and grief that he wasn't the same father I knew. But, he was happy and content. And, I realized the negative emotions were my issue to deal with.

After my father passed away, I found a calling to go back and volunteer at that place that had initially made me uncomfortable. I realized it had given him something none of us in the family could offer: friends, activities and a place where he felt totally comfortable surrounded by others with similar issues. And, it allowed my mother to have time off for herself.

I started a painting program with an artist friend, putting to use the ten years of art classes I had taken. The program has since blossomed to include acrylic, watercolor and mixed media classes. I have watched with amazement at how these individuals with dementia, many of whom have never painted before and can't remember what they had for breakfast, have found a new side of their brain to explore. I've been interested to see how these enthusiastic participants seem to be less inhibited and more willing to experiment, compared with many adults. The program allowed them to share their creative talents, not only with their families but also in art exhibits around Houston. Their work, seen in the painted doves that grace this book, is a testament to how those with dementia still have much to offer.

In addition to my volunteering, I have been fortunate to be able to use my professional background to work as the marketing director for Amazing Place for the last three years. It's been said there's nothing better than using your talents for good. I can attest that's been true for me. This work, where I have had more opportunities to interact with people with various types of dementia, has transformed my perspective on the disease and those affected by it.

I have witnessed firsthand how even though their minds may be changing, the participants still show an essential need to have meaning and purpose in their lives. In this safe place where labels and facades vanish, they develop unexpected friendships. And, in this stimulating program, they continue to demonstrate curiosity. Their lives have not ended; they are just different.

After my mother was diagnosed with dementia, I ended up receiving what I consider an unexpected gift. Our relationship, which had been filled with pain and resentment, transformed to one of acceptance and forgiveness. We were each finally able to say, "I love you," to one another. When I recounted the redemption we experienced to friends and at my mother's memorial service, the story seemed to resonate with others: this frightening disease that was robbing memories and changing behaviors had provided an avenue for grace in our tumultuous relationship.

I began to see the countless other ways the disease was offering lessons and illuminating grace for those who entered the doors of Amazing Place, and I began to discuss examples with my colleagues. As we thought back over the past twenty years, we recalled stories of the participants. While they confirmed what we intellectually knew about dementia—it affects entire families—these stories are not the sad stories that you would expect. They have a lovely poignancy: without denying the inevitability of the fading and ending of life, they bring what is most important in life vividly into focus.

It was hard to know just which stories to share here, because we have seen this important lesson imparted in so many ways. The following stories, along with the dramatic shift in my mother's and my relationship after dementia, represent many of the ways that this grace manifests:

- The woman who co-founded Amazing Place and served as an early executive director displays extraordinary courage as she faces the disease herself with honesty and grace.

- A remarkable young woman moves across country to be the primary caregiver for her grandmother with dementia for six months and learns invaluable life lessons.

- A family becomes closer, taking cues from their strong husband and father dealing with early onset Alzheimer's, and demonstrates what it means to have gratitude for each moment.

- A grandmother whose three siblings all have Alzheimer's, not surprisingly, also develops the disease. Now, living with her daughter and son-in-law who both work in the field of dementia, her grandchildren discover, early on, how to see the world through someone else's eyes.

- A caring social worker, who devoted her life to others, develops dementia and finds a way to continue to give back through her new-found artistic talent.

- A brilliant psychiatrist and his wife face the changes in his mind and eventual death with the ultimate peace and acceptance.

• A woman with dementia, who is beautiful inside and out, decides it is her ministry to bring joy to other participants at Amazing Place.

• Despite suffering from both Parkinson's and Alzheimer's diseases, a resilient woman demonstrates how her rock solid faith continues to anchor her.

• Three men from very different backgrounds have one thing in common—dementia—and they strike up a meaningful friendship.

As this unique program celebrates its twentieth anniversary, we saw an opportunity to provide understanding about dementia by sharing the faces and stories of those who are touched by it. These faces come from all walks of life, all ethnicities and all ages. Dementia doesn't discriminate. But more importantly, they demonstrate the power of faith and connection, the importance of acceptance and purpose, the value of mindfulness and gratitude and the resilience of those who have lost a portion of their brain but find another part to use.

Every day at Amazing Place, we witness how those with dementia still have much to contribute—whether it's their histories, or their laughter or their art. While it is many people's worst nightmare to lose their memory and part of their minds, our participants show us that in spite of these losses, their souls remain intact. Their lives can still have meaning. They can still teach us. And, when labels are stripped away, as they inevitably are with dementia, we are able to see these people for who they really are. There is nothing to hide behind: no masks, no material treasures, no bragging rights. What makes us valuable and human is what we can still see.

In this very special place—Amazing Place—this lesson of grace and inspiration became so visible to me and to others: we all are children of God, we are all equal, and we are all amazing in our own way. We trust these stories will help you, whether your life has been touched by dementia or not, to remember what truly matters.

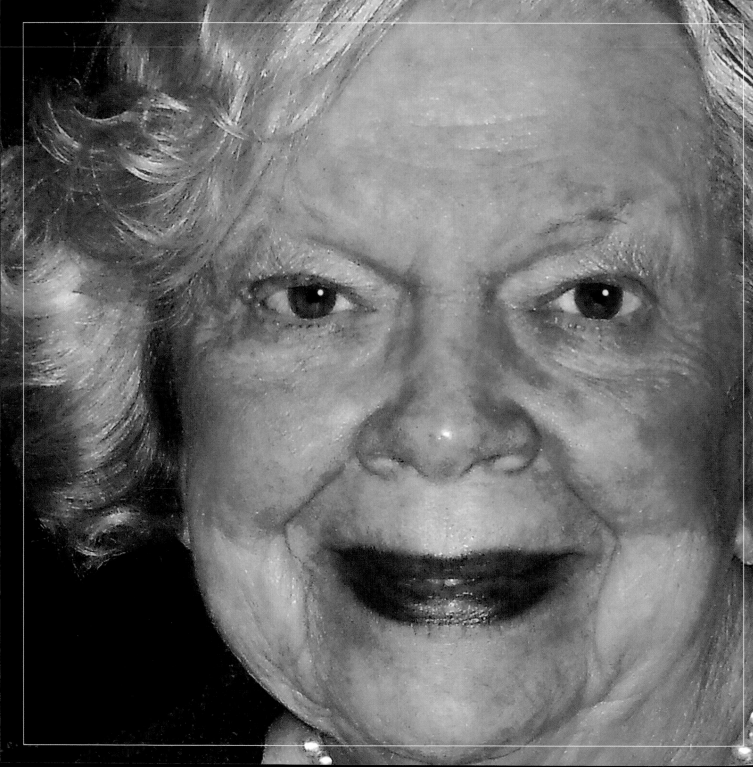

FORGIVENESS
A Relationship Transformed

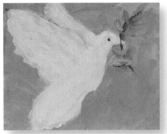

"Please let *me* do it, so I can call it my own," my mother spoke emphatically after I made the mistake of taking hold of her paintbrush. Sitting at my kitchen table, she was putting the finishing touches on a painting of a cerulean blue butterfly as she studied a similar image on my iPad. It reminded me of something my daughter might have said to me. I tried to be supportive and encouraging about her colors and composition. "I like your use of the green in the leaf against the blue butterfly," I said, without trying to sound condescending. I could feel she appreciated this time together, something she had always yearned for.

This tender scene would have been hard for me to imagine just a few short years before. That day, she was deep in her dementia, and I knew that it was not unusual for those with Alzheimer's to slowly regress. I was working on striking that delicate balance of maintaining her respect and dignity even as she acted more childlike. But what was most surprising about this scene was the contrast to our past relationship, which had been so complicated and tumultuous.

Growing up as the oldest of four siblings, I felt keenly resentful of her lack of attention. It felt like her focus was on what was going to make her happy—going back to school or a new career—but not necessarily her children. Our relationship continued a painful push-pull dance as an adult, each of us wanting something from the other we weren't able or willing to give. She had an insatiable need for time and attention, and it seemed whatever I did give was never enough.

After moving to Houston from New York, my husband and I would use a major part of our precious two weeks of vacation time to visit our families in New York each year. As we left, instead of saying "Thank you for coming," my mother would invariably ask, "So when are you coming back?" At family dinners when we were all together, we would take note of how quickly she would change the subject to be about her. Whether it was my daughter telling about her first day at camp or the latest play she was in, or my son talking about his lacrosse game, the conversation would turn into stories about how miserable she was at camp when she was just six, how she wrote and directed the

DEMENTIA OR ALZHEIMER'S?

For many, the terms dementia and Alzheimer's are interchangeable, but in reality, dementia is the umbrella term for a list of disorders (including Alzheimer's) that are characterized by cognitive decline severe enough to interfere with daily life.

Cognitive decline includes losses in memory, speech, judgment, reasoning, planning and thinking abilities.

Alzheimer's disease is the number one cause of dementia, accounting for 60 to 80% of cases of dementia.

More than 5 million Americans are living with Alzheimer's disease, 2/3rds of whom are women.

The 6th leading cause of death in the United States, Alzheimer's is the only disease among the top ten in the US which cannot be prevented, slowed or cured.

One in three seniors will die with Alzheimer's or another dementia.

Brain changes due to Alzheimer's may begin 20 years or more before memory loss appears.

As many as 1/2 of older adults with dementia have more than one cause, with the most common being Alzheimer's combined with vascular dementia.

All information in sidebars throughout the book is sourced from the Alzheimer's Association 2016 Alzheimer's Disease Fact and Figures. www.alz.org

Junior Show at college, or reciting a cheer from her cheerleading days. We'd all lock eyes with one another or kick each other under the table in recognition of her "all about her" stories, and smile. Despite knowing that her childhood with a depressed mother had contributed to her self-centeredness, I still longed for her to be a doting mother and grandmother.

In 2001, when she was recovering from small cell lung cancer, my father, who had been a successful marketing executive at an international pharmaceutical company, started showing signs of dementia after having a triple bypass. He was diagnosed with frontotemporal dementia (FTD), a type of dementia that affects executive function. A brilliant executive, he had now lost his ability to plan and organize. But, even more difficult to watch, he also was losing his social awareness and impulse control. In spite of diabetes and cardiac issues, he would think nothing of diving into a carton of ice cream any chance he had or cursing shamelessly. My parents' money was running low, and neither of them was capable of paying their bills. When my husband, Bob, took over their finances long-distance, he realized we needed to step in before their money ran out. It turned out that they hadn't been responsible in planning for retirement, so we encouraged them to move from New York to be closer to us in Houston. Between their health and financial issues, it was time to oversee their lives as well.

Initially, I had this fantasy that it would feel immensely gratifying to help "rescue" them, a fitting role as the eldest daughter. We didn't believe we would have much time with them, given the seriousness of their illnesses, but even our good friends thought this would be the opportunity for me to reconcile my relationship with my mother.

We found an apartment for them just a few blocks away from our house and helped them get settled into their new lives as Texans, after more than seventy years of being New Yorkers. A few years later, when we helped our son settle in at college, it felt strangely similar. We introduced them to our church, which helped their adjustment. My mother quickly developed new friends and found volunteer opportunities. Like many baby boomers, I was living out the classic "sandwich generation" role with a fifteen-year old and seven-year old at home, working as a marketing consultant, and now, feeling responsible for my parents.

The first nine years challenged me in ways I could not have imagined. From monitoring their medications and worrying about their health, to managing their finances, we were now on the front lines of caregiving with siblings who lived far away. What proved most difficult, however, was watching my mother's lack of attention to my father as he sunk into deeper dementia. It triggered my own memories of how she had always focused on herself, often to the neglect of her children.

As I soon learned, it's not unusual for a crisis to finally cause action when it comes to dementia.

One typically hot, humid summer day in Houston, my mother called, hysterical, and said, "Your father is missing and I can't find him!" We called the police, and then each of us headed out, searching streets and his favorite haunts—including the nearby Ben and Jerry's™ ice cream store. There was no sign of him. After a frantic few hours, someone from his favorite train store, Papa Ben's, called to say my father was there—a mile away. He had fallen in the middle of one of Houston's busiest streets, and a kind stranger had helped him up and led him to the store, where he said he was heading. At that point, we were finally able to convince my mother she could no longer leave him alone.

As I soon learned, it's not unusual for a crisis to finally cause action when it comes to dementia. That's when we found Amazing Place. It turned out be a wonderful haven for both my father and mother. He made some new friends, enjoyed drawing—a long dormant talent—and excelled at trivia games, as his memory, as is common with FTD, was intact. My mother had time for herself and received much-needed

DIAGNOSING DEMENTIA

It's often challenging to diagnose the specific type of dementia as symptoms may overlap.

Doctors will look at medical history, physical exam, lab tests, and changes in thinking and behavior to help diagnose the type of dementia.

Getting diagnosed as early as possible is beneficial for a number of reasons. It allows people to:

- **Explore treatments** earlier to maintain independence as long as possible.

- **Increase chances** to participate in a clinical drug trial.

- **Have more time** for the family to obtain support and plan for the future.

- **Determine if the dementia** symptoms are like those of 9% of older adults whose condition is potentially reversible and caused by:

  Depression

  Side effects of medication

  Excess use of alcohol

  Certain vitamin deficiencies

  Thyroid problems

emotional support from the staff. Knowing he was safe was a tremendous relief to all of us.

It wasn't long after my father died of heart and kidney issues that my mother started exhibiting signs of dementia herself. Like many families, in which siblings live out of town, it took time to get everyone to acknowledge the reality of what we were seeing. Even after she had a transient ischemic attack (TIA), there was skepticism. Some family members thought that it was chemo brain, or just a worsening of her spaciness. But as newspapers piled up in her apartment, she was getting lost driving, and she finally confessed that the fire department had been called a number of times due to her burning food, I made the appointment to see a neurologist.

Once she was diagnosed with a combination of vascular dementia and Alzheimer's, something profound happened in our relationship. It was almost like a switch flipped; I began to see her in a completely different light. I accepted that she was no longer the mother I knew, and could never be the mother I had longed for. I recognized that her behavior was no longer in her control.

What had once been hurtful and made me angry, now I found endearing. One day, while visiting her in her assisted living home with my nineteen-year-old daughter, my mother turned to her and exclaimed unabashedly,

"Tell me a story about me!" I teased her, but in a loving way, and we all laughed. I realized it was the first time she could laugh at herself. And instead of feeling indignant, I found it humorous.

On another occasion, with tears in her eyes, she painfully confided to me, "I just miss my mind." Now, instead of the resentment I had felt towards her for so long, I felt intense compassion. I was finally able to accept her self-focus and realize that she was just another wounded child, as we all are.

As her dementia deepened, we were both able to appreciate and acknowledge each other's strengths. I came to see her youthful vigor, creativity and lust for life with new admiration. I felt pride, like never before, for how uncommon it had been for a mother in the early sixties, to have so much ambition for a career and return to graduate school to become a guidance counselor. I learned to appreciate how hard it must have been for this native New Yorker to move to Texas after seventy years, and how seamlessly she had embraced Houston as her new home. And, I came to value her ability to hold on to her dreams, even in her dementia, including her goal of one day opening a beignet store.

When my mother was her most vulnerable and least inhibited, we found the relationship each of us had been searching for all those years.

She began to call me "her rock." For the first time, instead of complaining that I wasn't doing enough for her, she became effusive in her praise and grateful for our time together. It made it easier to be with her, and I looked for things to do with her that she would enjoy. One memorable day, I thought she'd love a makeover at a department store make-up counter. While I once would have never indulged her in her vanity, now it seemed a loving thing to do. It turned out to be entertaining as well. As she looked in the mirror and used her hands to pull back her face, she exclaimed cheekily to the saleswoman that what she really needed was a facelift. The woman laughed and said, "Well, we don't do that here!" I whispered to her that my mother had dementia, and the next thing my mother said was, "How about some eyebrows and eyelashes? Uggh, I look so old!" By this point, a few other sales people had gathered around and my mother adored the attention. They whispered back to me, "She's so cute!"

She started calling me and telling others I was her mother. I had become her advocate and protector, and she seemed to realize that. It felt somewhat ironic, as my whole life I had wanted her to be a better mother and felt she looked to her children to mother her. Now, she was acknowledging this dynamic, and I embraced the role I had once resented.

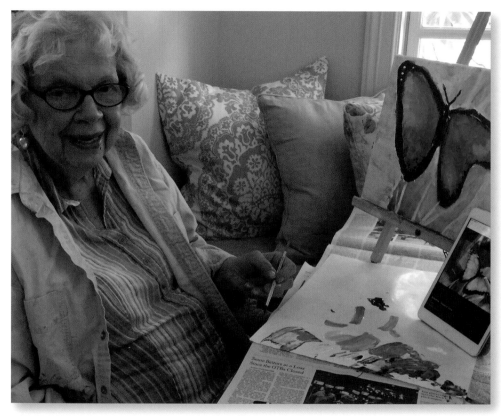

Each time we talked on the phone or I visited her, we would say to one another, "I love you." What is most surprising is that we had never uttered these simple words to each other before.

Several months before she died, I was sitting with her on her bed when her nurse, Amy, came in. Out of the blue, she bluntly confessed to Amy that she hadn't been a very good mother and even declared, "I was a bitchy mother." Even though I had searched for an apology for years, I tried to reassure her, saying, "Well I didn't turn out so badly!" She immediately responded, "That's because you had so much therapy!" It made me laugh; and she seemed surprised, as she was totally serious (and accurate). But I also realized in that moment that I was no longer angry and she was making amends in her own way.

When my mother was her most vulnerable and least inhibited, we had found the relationship each of us had been searching for all those years. Her dementia, which I originally had seen as taking away the opportunity for our relationship to improve, had given us the opportunity to forgive and accept each other.

Three months after she finished her butterfly painting in my kitchen, she passed away. We placed that painting, her last, in front of her ashes at her memorial service. She would have glowed knowing it was front and center and receiving so much attention. And maybe she did know.

Today, my life work is dedicated to those living with dementia and their families. It is clearly not a coincidence. I know it is my way to remain connected to her—a mother I once thought I would never be close to. Her butterfly painting sits on my desk at Amazing Place—a fitting reminder of how our relationship miraculously transformed. All because of dementia.

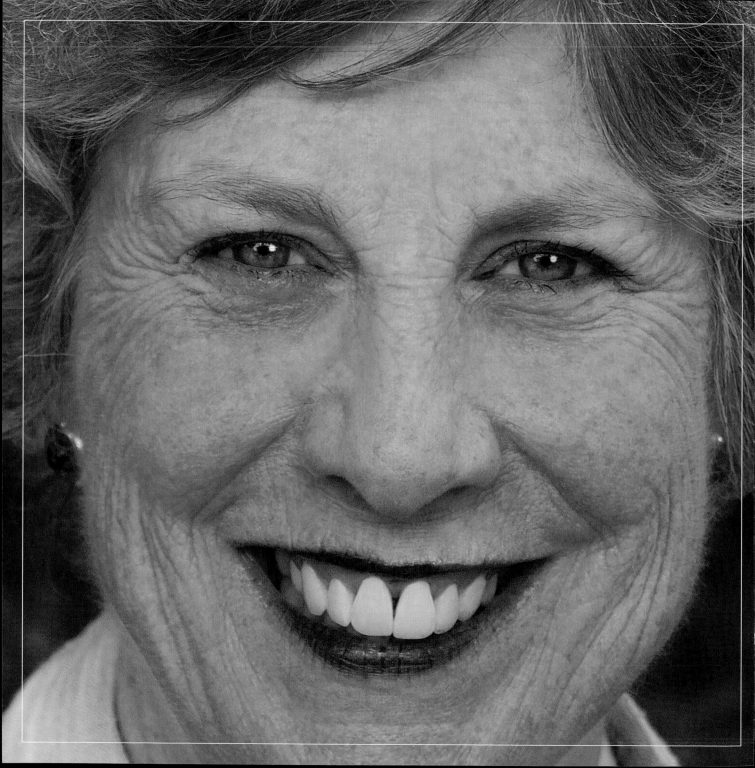

COURAGE

Facing the Truth Head-On

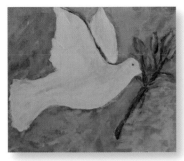

It's not unusual for someone who begins to notice memory issues to hide it, deny it, compensate for it or let family and friends cover for it. But for Margaret Bandy, whose life work revolved around serving those with dementia, there was no option but to embrace it.

Margaret has always been known as a forthright person. She tells it like it is. Ron, her husband of almost fifty years, says that Margaret—Missy, as he calls her—developed a tough skin growing up with an alcoholic father who caused them to move around a lot as he lost multiple jobs and died at only fifty-four. But as Ron says, no matter what adversity she faces, she is always upbeat and never complains. He refers to it as "The Missy Spirit." These attributes have served to support and strengthen Margaret throughout her life, and especially today.

Having had a mother who had early-onset "senility" in her early sixties, before the terms Alzheimer's or dementia were prevalent, Margaret was well aware of the warning signs. She had moved her mother from Dallas to Houston so she could supervise her care. Eventually, her mother was diagnosed with Alzheimer's disease, and Margaret had an intimate view of the impact and progression of the debilitating disease. She visited her mother almost every day until she died, close to twenty years from the time of her early diagnosis.

For Margaret, dementia care soon became a life mission. She had raised her three children, a son and two daughters, and worked as an English, bible and art history teacher. Her youngest daughter, Liz, says Margaret was "a multi-task, take-charge mother who could balance work and family and also be president of the PTA." Knowing Margaret's experience with dementia, her pastor, Rev. Dean Robinson, the visionary pastor of Senior Ministries at St. Luke's Methodist, asked her to help develop a program to assist the growing numbers of families who were facing the challenges of a loved one's memory loss. It was the early 1990s, before many support services existed, and Margaret chaired the founding committee to research and plan for an innovative day program. The group saw it as a way to provide a safe and stimulating place for those with memory issues and to provide support and well-deserved respite for the caregivers. Two years later, in 1996, The Seniors Place Adult Day Center, which would change its name to Amazing Place in 2009, opened in the church with Margaret as president of the Board. Within a year, she was serving as its executive director.

As the program grew and twelve churches joined to support the organization, it moved to a stand-alone building to accommodate the increasing numbers of participants. Not long thereafter, Margaret realized something was not right. She was only sixty-two, but she noticed she wasn't as organized as she used to be. She says she realized she was making mistakes that were not normal for her and wasn't remembering things like she should. Even though others failed to notice the subtle changes, including Ron, she insisted on seeing a doctor. Knowing the top neurologists in town through her work, she made an appointment to be tested. With a diagnosis of mild cognitive impairment (MCI), she matter-of-factly went to the Board and said, "It's time to find a replacement. I have dementia." She recommended Tracey Brown, the community liaison she had hired and mentored, to become the new executive director, and the Board agreed.

She is quick to acknowledge she has dementia, with no shame.

That was 2005. Since then, Margaret was put on medications, and her decline has been gradual. When she noticed she was losing her sense of direction, she made the decision to stop driving. Today, she has a harder time making decisions, like what to wear, and forgets from moment to moment what was said. Once, the life of the party and the hostess to whom everyone gravitated, it's now harder for her to initiate conversations.

Recently, it was clear to Ron that Missy needed more activity and social stimulation. He mentioned the idea of going to Amazing Place—where she still served on the Advisory Board and Tracey was still executive director—this time as a participant. She didn't flinch, and today, she says how happy she is to be there, albeit in a very different position. Margaret attends two days a week with participants who have a range and varying degree of symptoms, depending on where they are in the progression of their type of dementia. Her symptoms are still on the milder side. Margaret enjoys bridge, exercise and social interactions, sitting with the same group of women at lunch each day she attends. One of her tablemates, who suffers from vascular dementia, was a participant when Margaret was executive director. It doesn't seem to faze either of them that now they are on the same side of the table. One of the first staff members Margaret hired, David Mendoza, still works as a program leader leading exercise, sometimes for his former boss.

When asked, Margaret is more than happy and proud to tell the story of the beginnings of Amazing Place. Ron, too, is benefitting from the program she once led, as he has attended caregiver support groups to share his feelings of sadness and grief and learn that he's not alone.

Ron says Missy's strength continues and she never complains or asks, "Why me?" even when she faced a recurrence of breast cancer shortly after going back to Amazing Place. She had to begin several trying rounds of chemo-therapy, lost her hair again, and was unable to attend Amazing Place for a few months. Fortunately, she is in the clear with her cancer and is back as a participant, albeit not happy with her now curly "chemo" hair.

Margaret is quick to acknowledge she has dementia, with no shame. When asked how she keeps her positive attitude, she responds with a litany of sayings and a tad of indigna-tion—"Worry doesn't do any good." "That's not the way I do business." "What doesn't kill you makes you stronger."

When it is suggested that her honesty about her diagnosis is both unusual and inspiring, she contends, "Knowledge is something to stand on. If you embrace it, it's no longer the enemy."

Her adult children also find her strength remarkable, even as they mourn the loss of the strong mother she once was. "It's a circle of life event," says Griff, the eldest, who has four children with his wife Lisa and lives within a few miles of his parents. He's clearly referring

NORMAL AGING VERSUS DEMENTIA

Many people wonder if their memory changes are age-related or caused by dementia. Below are some examples of the differences:

NORMAL AGING		SIGNS OF DEMENTIA
Missing a monthly payment	vs	Inability to manage a budget
Forgetting which day it is and remembering later	vs	Losing track of the date or season
Sometimes forgetting a word	vs	Difficulty having a conversation
Losing things from time to time	vs	Misplacing things and putting them in unusual places
Making a bad decision once in awhile	vs	Poor judgment, like writing large checks to telemarketers
Occassionally needing help to record a TV show	vs	Difficulty driving to a familiar location or remembering rules of a favorite game

For Ron, there is understandable sadness at watching his vibrant, intelligent wife slowly lose her memories.

to the way his mother faces the disease her mother had for so many years and for whom she carried the load of caregiving. He recognizes how his mother continues to be a role model, demonstrating how to handle adversity with grace and dignity. "She's always been a godly woman and never lets it get her down. She just takes it as it comes, even knowing what lies ahead."

Margo, the middle daughter who lives in Dallas, acknowledges it's sometimes hard because she sees her mother in intense spurts for a few days at a time, which makes the changes more noticeable. She worries about the toll it's taking on her Dad, recognizing how hard it is for him, but notices how it's her mother who continues to encourage him. She says watching old family videos makes it even more poignant as you realize "how she was such a take-charge person and how that's changed." She notes how her mother will reassure the family, saying in her straightforward style, "Well, we're all going to die of something."

Liz, the youngest daughter who also lives in Houston, adds, "Mom never shies away from talking about her illness and will even remark that between her brother and her, she 'drew the black bean.'" Like the rest of her family, she claims her mother's fighting spirit, or "Missy spirit," keeps her going. Since Liz was the child still at home while Margaret

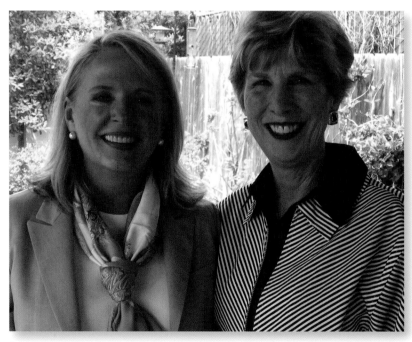

Margaret with Tracey Brown, her replacement as Amazing Place Executive Director, 2005.

devoted so much time to caring for her grandmother, she says that she learned through her mother's example how to deal with someone with dementia, skills she can use now with her mother.

For Ron, there is understandable
sadness at watching his vibrant,
intelligent wife slowly lose her
memories. He says it's hard when
friends seem to think she's doing
fine and don't realize the reality at
home. He acknowledges, "I thought
I was strong, but I realized I needed
help." But he also is supremely
grateful for the resilient woman
he married who now attends the
program she helped found, the
person who is candid about her
disease and never feels sorry for
herself, even now. She just moves
on. "I thank the Good Lord that
she's so happy to be there. I know
she doesn't tell you something she
doesn't mean. She gives *me* courage."

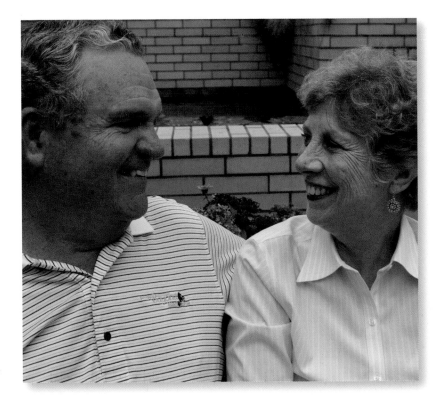

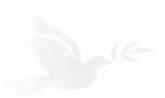

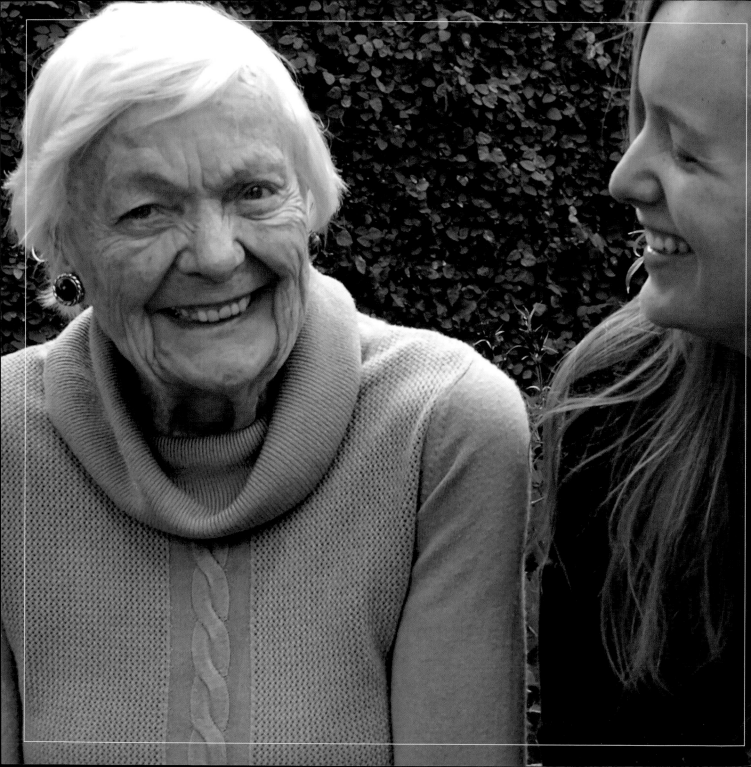

AUDACITY

Bridging the Gap

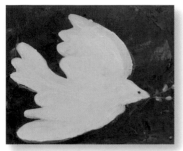

A fresh-faced young woman with long, straight blonde hair, looked like she was still in college. She stood out amongst the mostly middle-aged caregivers, many dressed in their holiday sweaters or red dresses, at the annual Holiday Tea held at Amazing Place. It was an event intended to support the spouses and adult children who carry the load of caregiving for their loved ones with dementia. But, this twenty-seven-year-old woman *did* belong there. Kelley Ruhl had just moved across the country to Houston, leaving behind two jobs and her life in Portland, Maine, to become the primary caregiver for her grandmother Mary Ruth Chelton, whose dementia was progressing.

Growing up in the small town of Lincoln, Maine, Kelley had an adventurous and caring spirit. While earning her degree in social work, she studied abroad in Russia and Australia and then worked as an au pair in Germany. After two years with the Peace Corps in South Africa, where she taught nutrition, hygiene and AIDS prevention to staff and at-risk children at an HIV/AIDS community center, she headed back to Maine to be closer to family. There, she pursued two of her passions, working as a doula and a baker. Her days included experiences as varied as holding the hands of a Burundian refugee woman during a forty-four-hour labor and waking at four each morning to walk to Love Cupcakes where she mixed batches of cupcake batter and witnessed customers' enjoyment of the final product.

Kelley had known her grandmother, "G-ma", much the way many grandchildren whose extended families live far apart know them—from family reunions, holidays and occasional family vacations. She described her grandmother as sassy, independent, and generous. Mary Ruth had devoted her life to raising her four children as the family moved around the country with her husband who worked for Texaco, ultimately landing in Texas.

Family was always her first priority—including doting on her nine grandchildren and three great grandchildren. When the grandchildren who lived in her neighborhood were younger, they would often hang out at their G-ma's house after school. As a widow for over thirty years, she grew her own vegetables, managed her own investments and was known as a card shark. She also worked tirelessly as a volunteer and was committed to helping those less fortunate, especially the homeless.

A few years ago, Mary Ruth, who lived alone, claims she felt "something let go" in her head. Suddenly, she could no longer drive, pay her bills, answer the phone, or remember to eat. Recognizing the clear signs of dementia—what they eventually learned was vascular dementia—her four adult children decided together that Janice, the sister who lived in Houston, would move in with her. However, when

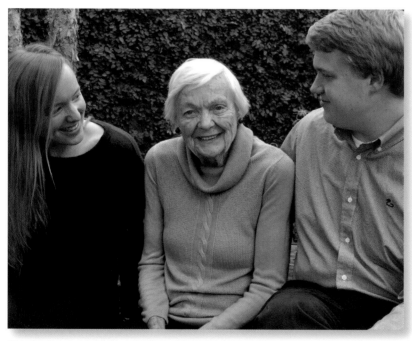

Mary Ruth with grandchildren, Kelley and Casey, at Amazing Place.

Mary Ruth went to visit her other daughter, Kelley's mom Jeannette, in Lincoln last summer for a few months, it became obvious that she needed even more supervision than Janice, who worked full time, could provide. She needed prompting to eat, bathe and do most anything.

Moving her to the cold winters in Lincoln with few resources for support or having Jeannette move to Houston and leave her husband behind didn't seem like good options. But, in a selfless and bold offer, Kelley volunteered to make the move herself to care for her grandmother and to help find her a more permanent living solution that was safe and appropriate. Kelley felt it was one more door that would open to uncharted territory, to teach her, and one more opportunity to care for someone in need. And that energized her.

While Kelley had worked with children and adults in her previous social worker roles, being the primary caregiver for a family member with dementia posed very different challenges. While she supervised her grandmother's daily activities—ensuring she ate, showered and dressed—Kelley acknowledged, "It felt surreal at first, as I was doing the same things for her that she had done for my mother and me." Initially, her grandmother was reluctant to accept her young granddaughter's role as caregiver. Kelley added, "Sometimes, it was like working with a toddler who had ninety years of attitude!"

In her role, she also oversaw her grandmother's medical care, consulting as needed with her mother, including managing medications, choosing doctors, scheduling and taking her to appointments and deciding on surgeries. Just as importantly, she became astutely aware of her grandmother's mental and emotional health, including keeping her engaged and happy. Kelley got an inside view of the caregiving role where the work day is twenty-four hours a day, seven days a week. She noted something many other caregivers feel: "I found it hard to separate my work day from the rest of my life".

> Kelley saw this time as a chance to truly get to know her grandmother—her loves, her interests, her history.

Being the resourceful person she was, Kelley soon found Amazing Place. She felt it was an ideal place for her grandmother to go a couple of days a week, for socializing and stimulation, while giving her some time off. There, Mary Ruth could be around others her age with similar memory issues and also engage in activities like playing cards and exercising. On the days she attended, Kelley noticed how her grandmother became much more alert and present. "She would look you in the eye and participate in conversations again." Although Kelley didn't initially know it, Mary Ruth also had a couple of coincidental connections with Amazing Place. She had volunteered for years helping the homeless with founder Rev. Dean Robinson. And, in a truly serendipitous twist, one of her grandsons, Casey, who had recently graduated with a degree in psychology, began his first real job as a program coordinator there, shortly after she started.

Kelley took her new role seriously, much like a devoted mother. She went to extraordinary lengths to find things to do that challenged but neither frustrated nor insulted her grandmother. They carved pumpkins at Halloween, used her grandmother's button collection to make Christmas ornaments and played Uno. When Kelley learned that her grandmother loved wildflowers, she found a game of Wildflower Bingo for them to play together. On the days she wasn't at Amazing Place, they went to the library to look for books on birds or short stories. Each Wednesday, they would head to lunch at Lucky's, a restaurant where one of Mary Ruth's other granddaughters worked.

OTHER TYPES OF DEMENTIA

Different types of dementia are connected with the region of the brain where brain cell damage occurs. In Alzheimer's, the hippocampus, which is the center for learning and memory is first impacted, which is why memory loss is one of the earliest symptoms.

Some of the other types of dementia include:

Mild Cognitive Impairment (MCI) – a slight, but noticeable decline in cognitive abilities, with an increased chance of developing Alzheimer's or another dementia.

Vascular – the second most common type accounting for approximately 20% of cases, occurs after a stroke that blocks brain blood vessels.

Frontotemporal dementia (FTD) – affects executive function and inhibitions.

Dementia with Lewy bodies (DLB) – similar symptoms as Alzheimer's disease, but sleep disturbances, hallucinations and gait imbalance also often occur.

Mixed dementia – a combination of dementias such as vascular and Alzheimer's.

Parkinson's disease – as Parkinson's progresses, it often results in dementia similar to Lewy bodies or Alzheimer's.

Normal pressure hydrocephalus – symptoms include difficulty walking, memory loss and inability to control urination.

While Kelley admits this time had its stress, it was also extremely gratifying. She saw firsthand how her efforts made a concrete difference in her grandmother's life. "She was less confused, isolated and irritable. And, she started eating better and was more social." While her grandmother clearly benefitted from the care and attention Kelley provided, Kelley saw this time as a chance to truly get to know her grandmother—her loves, her interests, her history.

"I've gone through a treasure chest with her of old letters and photos and learned about stories I didn't know about my family. I've relived history looking at newspaper clippings she kept on the moon landing and JFK assassination. I had a chance to read her wedding announcement and letters she wrote to her own mother. I learned about her friendship with a famous artist in Houston, her button collection and her love of owls!" Kelley also learned about dementia. "Before this, I didn't understand how dementia worked and how it can limit your patience."

Since part of Kelley's mission was to find a place for her grandmother to live permanently after she left, she spent a lot of time researching care options in Houston. After narrowing it down to two assisted living facilities, Kelley had her mother Jeannette, come down to finalize the decision and help Mary Ruth make the big move, leaving her home of almost twenty years.

After six months under Kelley's care, Mary Ruth transitioned smoothly to her new home. While Kelley says her grandmother now doesn't seem to remember the months they spent together, it doesn't bother her. "After all, that means she's not looking back and is happy where she is. I think my job is complete!"

Jeannette is immensely grateful for her daughter's time with her mother. "It was a gift to my mother, our family and me." She says at first she was surprised that Kelley was willing to do it, but she realized Kelley saw an opportunity to help out the family. She adds, "Kelley has always felt the world's pain and immersed herself in helping others. I can remember one time when she was nine, looking out the hotel window in New Orleans, with tears streaming down her face, as she watched some daycare children sitting on the ground in a fenced-in basketball court, and she cried, 'Oh Mommy, they have no place to play!'"

According to Jeannette, Mary Ruth taught her the importance of doing something of substance in your life, something that mattered. Jeannette says she passed on the notion of "providing good soil to let your children grow."

Mary Ruth passed on the notion of "providing good soil to let your children grow."

Kelley's willingness to change the course of her life for six months inevitably changed her life and her grandmother's life for good. But it also shows how Mary Ruth's message got passed through the generations. Kelley Ruhl's loving actions remind us of the value of taking risks and looking beyond the fear of the unknown—at any age. When you do, you have the chance, just like Kelley did, to test your character and make a difference in the world and in yourself.

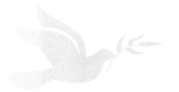

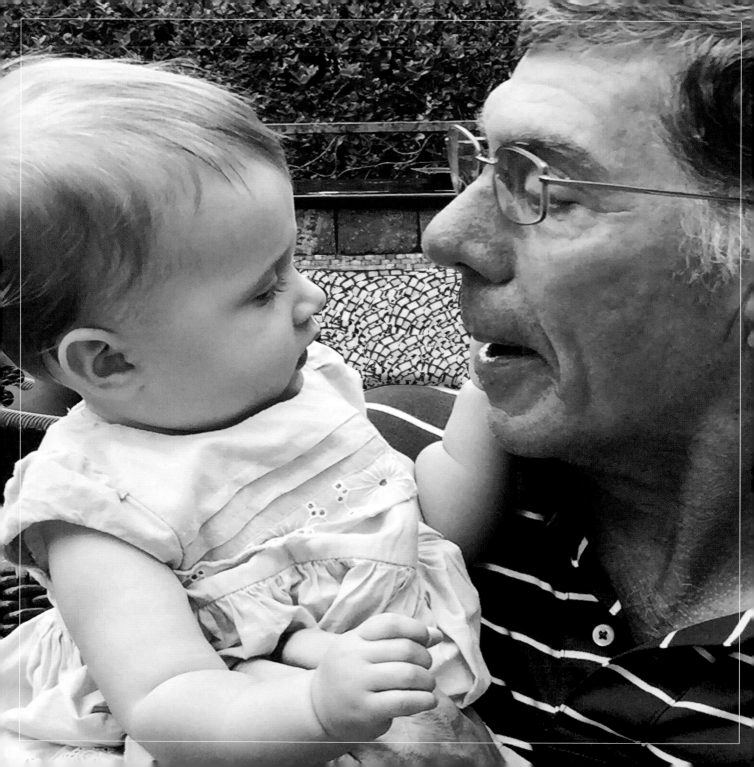

GRATITUDE
The Art of "Struggling Pretty"

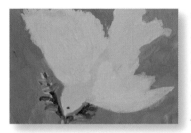

"I'm sorry to tell you—you have Alzheimer's." It's hard to imagine more terrifying words from your doctor, especially at the age of fifty-seven. But that's exactly what Jeff and Lisa Davis heard after Jeff went in for a sleep apnea test, followed by various neurological tests. Those words forever changed the lives of Jeff and Lisa and their daughters, Katelyn, Allie and Becca.

Jeff, a tough and successful attorney with a quick mind and wit, noticed he was having trouble preparing for a trial. Lisa was trying to figure out her next step in life, after their daughters left the nest for college. The only change in Jeff that Lisa had observed was that he had started handing her the check at restaurants to figure out the tip. She soon learned that difficulty managing money is a common early sign of dementia.

Their story is not so much about *what* happened to Jeff, but more about *how* he and his family have faced, "the cards he was dealt," as he described the situation at the time. And how, for these last nine years as his early-onset Alzheimer's has slowly changed the mind and behaviors of the husband and father they knew, the Davises have managed to find extraordinary gratitude.

While his family took the news of his diagnosis with understandable shock and grief, Jeff faced it with acceptance and reassurance. Serious, quiet and pragmatic, he was always the supportive father his daughters would call for advice. As was typical for the dad who was always in charge, he told them that there was nothing that could be changed; he would continue to live life as best he could and wanted them to continue to focus on their lives. According to Becca, who had just left for college at the time of his diagnosis, "When I offered to move back home, my dad said, 'Don't worry about me. I just want you to live out your dreams.'" Neither angry nor depressed, he worked to get things in order while he was still able. His daughters never heard him complain.

Over the years, as his memories have faded, the losses have mounted. Jeff had to prematurely retire, giving up his career of over thirty years. Then, it was handing over his car keys, which he did without hesitation realizing the liability issues if he continued to drive. More recently, Lisa found him about to use his razor to brush his teeth.

Lisa had to switch roles with Jeff, returning to work full time as a paralegal at Exxon Mobil. It was bittersweet, as it was this same role she had when she first met Jeff at a law firm where he was her supervisor. "I wasn't sure what I'd do next after the girls left home, but life happened, and it gave me a new role—taking care of Jeff like he did so well for our family all those years." Her plate is clearly full with her full-time position and the responsibilities of being Jeff's caregiver and the emotional support for the family.

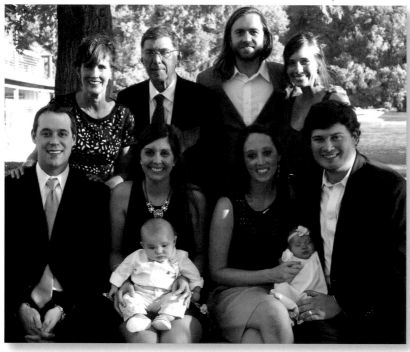

The Davis family, 2014, grateful for each moment.

She found Amazing Place to support both of them—as a program for him to stay social and active while she went to work. It was there that the beginnings of a different Jeff evolved as he explored a newfound passion for painting. The painting class was a new offering at Amazing Place and Jeff jumped in with enthusiasm. While his verbal skills diminished, his artistic side flourished. When he painted, his teachers noticed how he was especially calm and resolute. He always knew exactly what colors he wanted to use, often favoring bright hues in bold abstract designs. Each time he finished a composition, his eagerness to bring it home made his pride and accomplishment obvious. The more than forty abstract paintings he created at Amazing Place now adorn the walls of the Davises' home, as well as those of their daughters and a few special friends—gifts they will always treasure.

As the disease has progressed over the years, Jeff has become more dependent on others. Lisa is there, before and after her workday, to help him with bathing, shaving, brushing his teeth and getting dressed. She has adapted to the idea this is a different man than she married. She admits it's strange sometimes because he looks so healthy on the outside, typical of many with dementia. She's also learned to pay a lot more attention to taking time for herself, whether it is exercising, having dinner with friends or going on a long weekend away every few months. "It makes me better when I'm with him," she says.

Dealing with the losses of seeing Jeff diminish has only made this tight-knit family stronger as they lean on each other for support. Lisa, the "rock" of the family, contends that through prayer and her faith, she believes in her heart that God gave this to them to deal with for a reason. "I guess it is to teach me patience. And it's been an opportunity to show our daughters how to deal with adversity. I truly believe God only gives you what you can handle."

While the daughters all admit to processing their grief differently, they stay in close touch with each other, and especially with their mother. Katelyn, the eldest, notes, "She's trying to support everyone else, so we worry about who's supporting her." None of them have friends who are dealing with the same situation, which makes them feel it's hard for others to truly understand how they are slowly losing their father but have him still here.

What they all do have in common is an extraordinary ability to find the gratitude in each

EARLY-ONSET ALZHEIMER'S

If an individual younger than 65 has Alzheimer's disease, it is considered early-onset or younger onset Alzheimer's.

Up to 5% of those who have Alzheimer's have early-onset.

People can be diagnosed as early as their 40s or 50s.

Getting an accurate diagnosis is often challenging since doctors are not expecting it in younger people.

It is particularly challenging for these individuals as they may still have children at home, have careers or even be caregivers themselves.

Most cases of early-onset Alzheimer's are inherited, with a parent or grandparent who also developed the disease at an earlier age.

It's important to plan for the future when the disease is in its earliest stages.

Support groups are especially beneficial for those with early-onset Alzheimer's and their family members.

moment and appreciate what they still have. As Lisa says, "I don't focus on what I've lost as much as the small moments like when he beams with joy as he holds his two grandchildren. It's a wonder to see our granddaughter, Annaleigh, just sixteen months old, instinctively go over to him and pat him or put her head in his lap. It's something she would never do with me, and it's like she knows he needs special care."

Sharing what it was like to tell her dad she was pregnant with her second child, Katelyn adds, "How many friends can say they get to tell their father over and over that he's going to be a grandfather, and it's like the first time each time?" She acknowledges while he's not the grandfather she pictured, "I enjoy watching his face light up like a child when he gets on the ground to play with Davis, his grandson." She says she tries to take a lot of pictures to hold on to those moments.

Perhaps the most profound lesson they've each learned from Jeff's illness, is what the illness itself teaches by its nature.

"I lost the Dad I knew who raised me, but I have a new dad. He was more serious before, and now he is always happy," notes middle daughter Allie. "He danced all night at my wedding, something he would never have done before. And we all get a kick out of watching him laugh at silly movies now." She, too, is grateful for the memories she will have of her father playing with her young daughter, even though she knows her daughter may not remember those times.

Becca recently had the chance to live at home with her parents for a month which gave her an inside view of what her father is like day-to-day and her mother's amazing strength and patience. With her father talking less and less, she says, "His gestures mean all the more to me now. He will put his arm around my shoulder or motion for me to go on a walk with him. I've learned to appreciate those small moments." She adds that her mother's fortitude in taking on the roles of caregiver and provider in addition to loving wife, has been a model for her own marriage and the commitment to her wedding vows—in sickness and in health.

Perhaps the most profound lesson they've each learned from Jeff's illness, is what the illness itself teaches by its nature. By losing past memories, Jeff no longer has regrets; with no sense of the future, anxieties about what could happen disappear. As Lisa says, "Life is obviously much simpler for Jeff." No wonder Jeff is more contented. It's what programs about mindfulness teach—being aware and grateful for each moment. Jeff's family has taken this lesson to heart as they recognize each day with their father is a gift.

A couple of years ago, as Becca's husband, Kyle, one-half of the singer/songwriter duo, Penny and Sparrow, was writing his second album, "Struggle Pretty," he thought of Jeff. "The theme of the album," Kyle says, "is that we all face struggles, but the measure of a person's character is whether they face those tough times with grace or not. The valleys are inescapable. You can't always be on top of the mountain." The first song on the album, "Jeffrey Alan," was written in his father-in-law's honor, and when it came time to design the album cover, it made perfect sense to use one of Jeff's abstract paintings.

Jeff's art, the cover of the Penny and Sparrow album, "Struggle Pretty."

While the future is unknown, each one of the Davises will continue to "struggle pretty." They remind us all of the power of gratitude. As Becca said, "I just want to find joy in each little thing—even the tiniest speck."

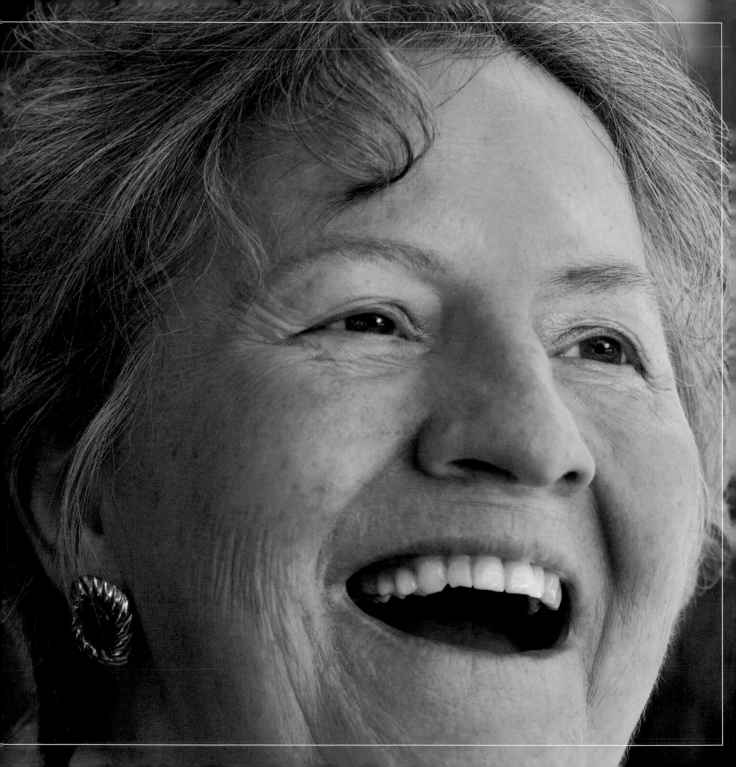

EMPATHY

Children Learn What They Live

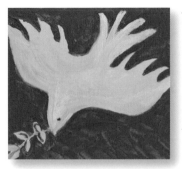

When Lois Drake started showing clear signs of dementia at the age of sixty-two, it was no surprise to her two daughters. She was now one of four of the five siblings in her family who had Alzheimer's disease. Her brother, the only sibling who hadn't been diagnosed with it, had died at the very young age of forty-two from a heart attack.

A neurologist confirmed that all four siblings carried the APOE-e4 gene—a gene that increases the risk of developing the disease, and at an earlier age. The news, while not totally unexpected, was obviously daunting, particularly for the potential implications for the next generation. But Lois' youngest daughter and son-in-law, Rachel and Emile, and their two children, Mia and Landon, with whom she now lives, have taken it all in stride. In fact, they now realize it's been a teachable moment for their family.

Lois and her siblings grew up fast after their father died of a heart attack at thirty-three. Lois was just five at the time, and her mother and the five kids moved from St. Louis to Houston to live with her Uncle Leo. He became a surrogate father to them, and they learned the importance of family. All the children worked from a young age to help support the family, including Lois, who started working at a downtown Houston movie theater at the age of eleven.

After marrying and having two daughters, Jennefer and Rachel, Lois continued to work until retiring ten years ago at the age of sixty. After she retired, she made a pact that she would take care of each one of her four grandchildren for their first year of life while her daughters worked. It gave her the chance to develop a special bond with each one while helping her daughters out.

Like her father, Lois' husband died at a young age, fifty-two, from complications of working at a chemical plant. It happened on a Thanksgiving weekend, and Thanksgivings were never the same for her after that. A number of years later, she decided she would save her money and take a few of her grandkids to Disney World during Thanksgiving week. It became a tradition from then on, and every other year or so, she would make the trek to "the happiest place on earth" with a couple of her grandkids. She loved it as much or more than they did.

In what seems a providential twist in retrospect, years before her mother had been diagnosed, Rachel had found her passion working with seniors who had dementia. While originally planning to be a physical therapist, during a college internship at a nursing home, she realized how much she loved hearing the stories of the seniors. She recognized that she could make the most difference in their lives as an administrator and has worked as a director in dementia-care facilities ever since.

In another coincidental twist, Emile also had a special interest and talent for working with seniors and those with dementia. For the last ten years, he has been the program director at Amazing Place, planning and conducting stimulating programs for those with mild to moderate dementia. He is known for his exceptional ability to communicate with those with dementia, redirecting them when needed and helping them to find things they can still do and enjoy.

Several years ago, signs started pointing to Lois' memory issues. She was repeating herself a lot. Then she totaled two cars, one flipping on a busy freeway. One day, while babysitting her grandkids, she forgot to pick them up from school. The final sign came when she fell while getting on an unsteady step-ladder to change a light bulb and broke her tibia, fibula, patella, humerus and shoulder. When Lois was diagnosed with mild cognitive impairment (MCI), Rachel knew her mother couldn't be alone anymore.

There was no hesitation in what she and Emile would do—Lois would move in with their family. "She was always so good to me and my children; now it was my turn to take care of

RISK FACTORS FOR ALZHEIMER'S DISEASE

Alzheimer's disease, according to experts, most often develops as a result of interactions among genes and other factors. **The three greatest risk factors** for Alzheimer's are:

Age – The greatest of the three factors is age, as most people with Alzheimer's are 65 or older. As age increases, so does the risk. One in nine people who are 65 or older and one in three who are 85 and older have Alzheimer's disease.

Family History – Those who have a parent or sibling with Alzheimer's are more likely to develop the disease, but it is not necessary to have a family history to develop the disease.

APOE-e4 Gene – Those who inherit the APOE-e4 form of the gene have an eight- to twelve-fold higher risk of developing Alzheimer's, but it is not guaranteed that they will develop Alzheimer's.

Other risk factors – While none of the above factors can be changed, research is showing that risk factors that can be managed through lifestyle and wellness choices include:

- Avoiding head trauma;
- Maintaining heart health through exercise and managing blood pressure, heart disease, diabetes and high cholesterol.

her," said Rachel. With two elementary-aged children, and working full time, she knew it was going to be a juggling act. As her mother's disease has progressed to Alzheimer's, Rachel says, "In many ways, it's like having another child to keep track of, but this one with more health issues and poorer judgment." It means more laundry, medications and doctor appointments. And, as it is for many with dementia who have diminished judgment, Lois's safety is more of a worry. She can't be home by herself, and she has to be watched constantly when the family goes out.

Both Rachel's and Emile's experience with dementia care has obviously been a help as they deal with her mother. Lois commutes with Emile every day to Amazing Place, where she enjoys playing bridge and doing art projects. She does not like to miss a day and is disappointed when Emile takes the day off and she can't go. "It's given them a special bond," says Rachel, who adds, "Now he can do no wrong." Emile modestly confesses that sometimes when Rachel is getting impatient, "I can divert Lois' attention and calm things down." They are good about reminding each other that the problem is not Lois, it's the disease.

Mia and Landon know not to say, "Don't you remember?" or "Mimi, you already said that."

For Lois, it's also been a plus to be with her grandkids. Rachel has noticed that her mom feels less impaired being with them and that she can still feel like she has a purpose when she helps out with them. She is very upfront about her memory issues and has been known to say when she can't remember something, "Oh, that stupid brain thing." She even will joke about it, saying things like "Oh, I better call my sister for her birthday, but if I don't, she won't remember."

Rachel and Emile are also demonstrating for Mia and Landon, who are twelve and eight now, how to deal with someone with dementia. Living with their grandmother, whom they call "Mimi," has matured them in ways they probably don't even realize. They have learned the delicate balance of being empathic and nurturing, while still preserving their grandmother's dignity. Even though there are times they are acting like parents to their grandmother—making sure she is safe, or bringing her something she's forgotten—they know how to do it without her realizing. They know not to say, "Don't you remember?" or "Mimi, you already said that."

In a reversal of the typical grandparent role, Lois will sometimes bring an art project home from Amazing Place and say, "I made this for Mia." And in a tender exchange, Mia will respond, "Oh Mimi,

I love it!" Mia says that the best room in the house is Mimi's where "she will braid my hair, we snuggle together on her bed and watch 'Dancing with the Stars.'" Even though she knows her grandmother keeps checking in on her all evening because she forgets she already has, Mia recognizes, "She does it because she loves me." She adds, "When we eat dinner and go around the table to talk about what made us happy today, Mimi says the same thing every night, 'I'm happy to be alive.'"

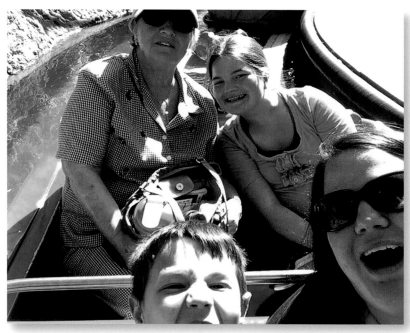

Lois, Mia, Rachel and Landon at Disney World for Lois's 70th Birthday.

Landon, too, has learned to be sensitive to Mimi and instinctively will go to reach for her hand in crowded places. When she forgets to get her drink, Landon will get it. Landon says he appreciates her going to his soccer games and bragging about him when he plays well. "Sometimes I have to remind Mimi that she already fed her dog, Ginger," he says, and he adds, "I like getting a kiss goodnight from Mimi if she doesn't fall asleep before me."

Rachel decided recently to celebrate Lois's seventieth birthday by taking her and Mia and Landon on a trip back to Disney World, Lois's favorite place. It was poignant to take her mom to the place she had always taken the grandkids. And, Rachel knew that it was probably the last time she could take Lois there.

It required a lot of special arrangements with the airlines and the parks to accommodate her mother. Rachel brought matching shirts for each day they were there, another way to make sure her mother didn't get lost. While Rachel acknowledged it was a lot of work, she said, "It was worth every moment to see her never stop smiling. It was like the first time she had ever been there, squealing with glee on the roller coaster." The kids understood the real reason they were there was for Mimi, so when she wanted to wait in a long line for pictures with Mickey, they didn't complain.

Rachel is asked all the time how she does it—working in the field of elder care, caring for a mother with dementia, and raising her two children. She acknowledges that her plate is full as wife, mother, caregiver and long-term-care administrator. This past fall, she had her own health scare—a heart attack. It was a wake-up call. The probability that she, too, could inherit Alzheimer's, is in her awareness as well. While most would obsess about it, Rachel is working on things she can control in her lifestyle—especially diet and exercise.

"When we eat dinner, Mimi says the same thing every night, 'I'm happy to be alive.'"

While she never regrets this time caring for her mother, she realizes there is another benefit she hadn't predicted: just as Lois learned early on from her mother and Uncle Leo the importance of taking care of family and passed that understanding to Rachel, now Rachel is passing it down to Mia and Landon.

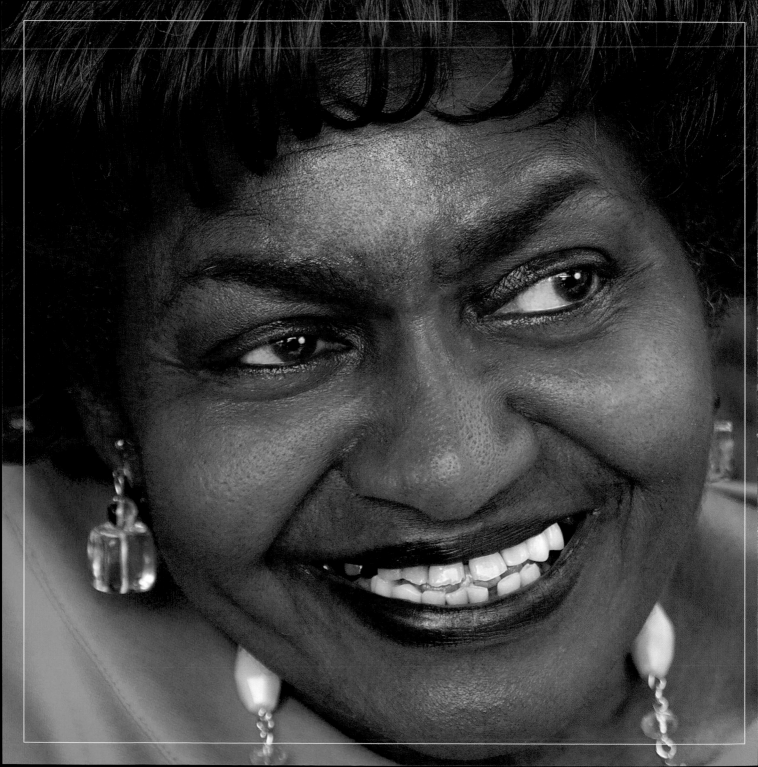

CREATIVITY
Discovering a New Side of the Brain

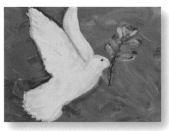

Gloria Carter's life has always been focused on giving to others. As a social worker for many years, she was the one who always took the cases others didn't want. As a single mother to two children, she always put their needs before her own. Now, as she experiences the losses associated with dementia, Gloria has discovered a new artistic talent which allows her to continue sharing her gifts with others.

When she was in her twenties, newly divorced and pregnant, Gloria moved back from California to her hometown of Houston with her two-year-old daughter, Yvette. She explains she had to leave a rough situation and was determined not to bring another child into the world to live with her husband. Her son, Phillip, was born soon after, and Gloria worked while she went back to college to get her degree and make a better life for them. Yvette remembers being a young child hanging out with her brother at the library while her mother studied. After she graduated, Gloria worked two jobs—as a social worker at Neighborhood Centers and a retail job at Foley's department store—while her mother and grandmother watched her children.

Soon after she started her social work job, Gloria noticed a pile of folders on her supervisor's desk and asked what they were. She was told that these were the cases no one wanted, as they required traveling all around South Texas to pick up sick children and take them to the doctor. At that moment, Gloria realized her mission was to take on these cases, determined to develop trust and relationships with these home-bound children and their parents. Gloria put her whole heart and soul into her work. She notes, "I always did things to make them comfortable like folding down the back seat to create a bed for them, bringing a special pillow with a pretty pillowcase for each one and playing soothing music."

In spite of Gloria's demanding workload, Yvette admits she spoiled her and her brother, even refusing to let them do chores. She always made sure they had plenty of clothes, while she owned just two pairs of pants—black and blue. One was always drying while she wore the other pair. It wasn't unusual for her to stay up all night sewing her daughter a new dress. According to Yvette, "We never felt like we were struggling, but we know she sacrificed so much for us."

A few years ago, after she had retired, unbeknownst to her children, Gloria initiated cognitive testing for herself. It surprised Yvette that Gloria hadn't shared her concern, but once she found out, she went with her to the neurologist and learned she had vascular dementia. The only dementia they were familiar with was Alzheimer's, but they discovered Gloria's dementia was a result of scarring on her brain, possibly from her high blood pressure. Unlike Alzheimer's, the decline has not been as progressive, although her memory and behaviors have definitely been affected.

ABOUT VASCULAR DEMENTIA

The second most common cause of dementia after Alzheimer's disease, vascular dementia happens when decline in thinking skills are caused by conditions that block or reduce blood flow to the brain.

Risk factors include age, smoking, diet, blood pressure, high cholesterol, weight, alcohol consumption and previous transient ischemic attack (TIA) or strokes.

Not all strokes result in vascular dementia, as it depends on the stroke's severity and location.

After a major stroke, sudden changes in thinking and perception may include confusion, disorientation, trouble speaking or understanding speech and vision loss.

Multiple small strokes or other conditions that affect blood vessels and nerve fibers deep inside the brain may cause more gradual thinking changes as damage accumulates.

Common early signs of widespread small vessel disease include impaired planning and judgment, uncontrolled laughing and crying, declining ability to pay attention, impaired function in social situations, and difficulty finding the right words.

Vascular dementia often occurs with other types of dementia, including Alzheimer's and Lewy bodies.

Gloria and her children have stayed unusually positive throughout her illness. Like many family caregivers dealing with dementia, Yvette acknowledges it's like having a new mom. "It's just a different season, and I've grieved the mom I used to have."

Gloria's neurologist recommended she attend an adult day program to keep her active. They found Amazing Place, where, in art classes, she has revealed a whole new side and developed an unexpected interest and passion for painting and other art pursuits. "It was quite a shock to see that it's the only thing she wants to talk about," says Yvette, who also says it's been a godsend in many ways. It gives Yvette something to ask Gloria about: "Have you finished any paintings?" "What are you painting now?" It also gives Gloria something to do with her at home, as Yvette has gotten her coloring books and markers. And, it's something Gloria feels good about and which she can share with others.

When asked why she enjoys art so much, Gloria says, "Art is something that is your own. No one else can do it like you. You use your own mind to paint what you want. It just makes me feel happy and calm. And it's something I can still do for my son and daughter."

Both children have benefitted from Gloria's prolific painting, with gallery walls of her work, often fighting over who gets a painting. "Now when I ask her to do a painting for me, I tell her to write my name on it!" says Yvette.

Gloria's artwork is distinctive, with a unique style of painting using vertical lines of color. She uses this same technique with her coloring books. Recently, Gloria decided she wanted to do a picture for her seven-year old neighbor, Skylar. When she gave it to her, Skylar was fascinated with Gloria's coloring style and wanted to learn how she did it. Now Gloria, at seventy-six and with dementia, is an art teacher, showing Skylar her technique. Yvette notes it's a perfect way for her mother to continue to give to others and adds that now friends are requesting that Gloria paint something for them too.

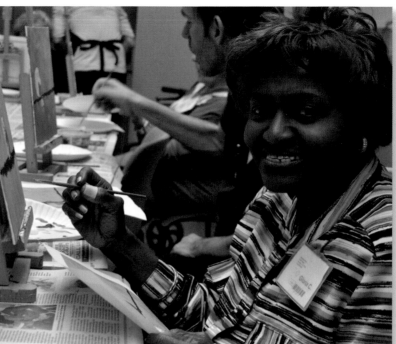

While it's hard to know if Gloria's creative talent is a result of, or in spite of, her dementia, what is clear is how it has enriched her life and the lives of others. Yvette is recognizing that while Gloria is not the same mother she knew, she can still embrace the new things about her mother. As Yvette notes, "Even in this season of her life, she can still contribute. I can still have a part of her. And it's something I'll have when she's not here anymore."

"Art is something that is your own. No one else can do it like you. You use your own mind to paint what you want."

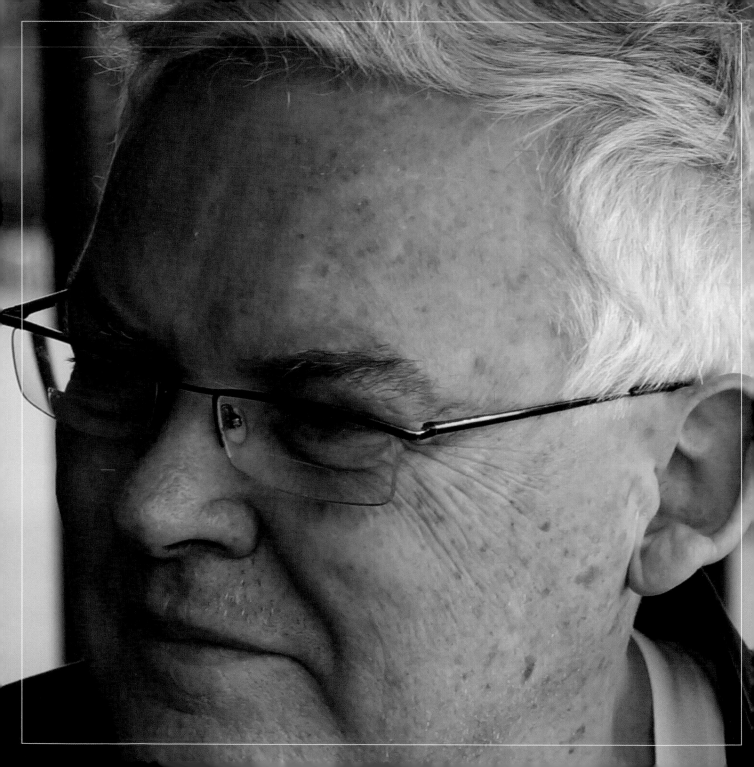

ACCEPTANCE

State of Mind

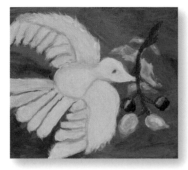

He was described as a gentle man. Humble, wise and inquisitive, Albert Ebaugh was a brilliant and prominent Houston psychiatrist who spent his life helping others to understand and manage their minds. When he learned he was gradually losing pieces of his own mind, it was a prime example of how dementia doesn't discriminate. But Albert showed how to accept this loss with amazing grace.

While he was dedicated to a life of helping others, his true love was his second wife, Helen Rose, with whom he loved to dance. They met fortuitously on a Sunday afternoon on a children's train ride at the Houston Zoo. A tall, striking man, Albert, recently divorced, sat in the last row of the miniature train with his two young sons. Helen Rose, a sociology professor and former nun, equally tall and attractive, was taking two young children of a friend of hers on an outing to the park. They sat in the seat in front of Albert and his sons. While she was trying to convince her young friends to go to the planetarium on the cold, December day, the dashing dad tapped her on the shoulder to ask about it. They chatted on the ride and the next thing they knew, the six of them headed to the zoo, where he bought everyone popcorn. Eighteen months later, Albert and Helen Rose married, and soon after, they added a daughter and another son to their family.

For over forty years, Albert practiced adult psychiatry at the top hospitals in Houston and earned the respect of his peers, serving as president of the Houston Psychiatric Society. He was also well regarded for his innovative use of hypnotherapy, before it was well known. His demeanor matched what one would expect in a psychiatrist—calm, reflective, kind. He was a man who listened with his heart.

After retiring in 2004, he began noticing he was having trouble with seemingly simple tasks like planning his day, filing his papers or placing the right pills in the right compartment of his weekly pill container. He felt frustrated at his incompetence with such mundane activities. Even Helen Rose, normally patient, was frustrated when he wasn't able to make plans for a trip or an evening out to the symphony. "I was finding myself getting mad that it was all on me," says Helen Rose in retrospect.

A brain scan confirmed what his geriatric psychiatrist suspected. Albert had frontotemporal dementia (FTD). Although Albert knew that it would rob him of executive function and judgment, but initially leave his memories intact, he took the news with a composed resignation. "It is what it is," he said. Helen Rose adds that the scan was actually a relief to her, an explanation for his changed behavior. "Once I saw it, in black and white, it helped me realize that I couldn't be angry at him for something he couldn't control."

From that moment on, he was pragmatic and realistic, determined not to be a burden to his family. referring to an assisted living facility in the neighborhood, he told Helen Rose, "If I get too much to handle at home and become a burden, just put me there." According to Helen Rose, he was never hard on himself and didn't fight the losses that came. "It was his decision to give up driving, realizing he didn't have the reflexes he once had....He wanted to maintain his respect."

"Death is not something you can avoid."

They learned about Amazing Place as a place for him to spend the day while Helen Rose continued to teach. During the three-and-a-half years Albert was a participant, he continued to use his relational and empathic skills, often offering free "counseling" to the other participants. He loved the diversity of the people and the opportunity to learn about their unique stories. "He would get in the car and go on and on about the different people he met that day, a federal judge, or a veteran, or an engineer," says Helen Rose. Most importantly, she said, he would talk about the respect and dignity that each person was given there. She adds, "He was so happy there. Amazing Place was a godsend and gave me the freedom not to worry."

When Albert started having issues with walking and other motor functions, not typical symptoms of FTD, his doctor gave him the stunning diagnosis. "You've got Lou Gehrig's disease. And you're going to die from this." Lou Gehrig's disease, or ALS, is often perceived as the antithesis of dementia, one that robs motor function as opposed to memories. Now his brain was being attacked from all sides. Albert's response was predictable. "Well, Helen Rose and I are going to die of something. Death is not something you can avoid."

His doctor encouraged them to begin hospice care. Albert wasn't sure if he would feel comfortable with someone in the house, but he ultimately acquiesced. They renovated a downstairs office into a bedroom for him; and hospice offered him medications to keep him comfortable and provided emotional support for both him and Helen Rose.

Soon after, on Easter weekend, he asked Helen Rose to have all the kids come over, as he wanted to talk to them. With his three sons and daughter gathered around his bed, he spoke lovingly to each one.

"Nelson, how proud I am of your career as a lawyer, but I'm most proud of what a good father you've been…keep doing what you're doing."

"James, can you believe I have a vascular surgeon as a son?"

"Sarah, I'm so grateful we had the time you lived with us after your divorce. We had a chance to reconnect. Just keep on going; you're going to be fine."

"Stephen, you've accomplished so much in your young life; but your biggest accomplishment is how you've balanced that with being a wonderful father to both your children."

There were tears as his children took his words to heart. Stephen tucked his three-month old daughter into the bed with his father. The family brought him anything he wanted, including dozens of tins of smoked oysters, his favorite, which piled up around his bed.

He wanted his family to be part of the dying experience. And, then, in the last three weeks, he started getting quieter, withdrawing. Helen

THE TOLL ON CAREGIVERS

More than 15 million Americans provide unpaid care for people with dementia.

83% of the dementia caregivers are family, friends or other unpaid caregivers.

Over 1/2 of these caregivers take care of parents, and 23% are "sandwich generation" caregivers.

Approximately 2/3rds are women, and over 1/3rd are daughters.

59% of family caregivers rate the emotional stress as high or very high.

Some of the recommended interventions for caregivers include:

Education about the disease and resources

Counseling

Support Groups

Respite—planned, temporary relief

Rose says she learned that dying is a lonely process, and you have to do it by yourself. "Our anxiety is we want to cling to them and not let them go. But when it's time, we have to let them go."

As he had in everything else, Albert took an active part in planning his memorial service. He chose a tender, reassuring passage by Max Ehrman, and his close friend read it.

"Be gentle with yourself.
You are a child of the universe,
no less than the trees and the stars.
In the noisy confusion of life,
keep peace in your soul."

As Albert desired, he was buried in his favorite, comfortable clothing—blue jeans—in a pine box lined in denim in Olfen, Texas. In this small West Texas community with a cemetery amidst the cotton fields, blue skies and wide open spaces, he felt most at home. He and Helen Rose had spent every Christmas for forty-one years here with her extended family. He handled his dying like he handled his life. He didn't fight it. He accepted it. He was at peace.

Fortunately, Helen Rose had learned the importance of taking care of herself from a caregiver support group at Amazing Place. She had started the process of building bridges to a future without him. After her soulmate and dance partner died, she continued to meet with her friends from the caregiver support group, joined a book club and started exercising at the YMCA. She admits spending the first week after his service sleeping, when a ninety-five year old friend advised her go the the gym and have some activity each day. She contends this prescription has been a salvation for her. She has also learned to be kinder to herself and forgive herself for the times she felt angry with Albert. And, finally, she says she tells others the importance of naming the disease and saying it aloud, without shame, "My parent/ husband/sister has dementia."

As Helen Rose shared in the months after his death, "His strength helped me deal with my grief. He was never scared of death. He was supportive of others till the end. He showed me how to die...and live. And that it's in moments you can't control when you find grace."

Albert's prayer card reads:

Hopi Prayer

Do not stand at my grave and weep.
I am not there, I do not sleep.
I am the thousand winds that blow.
I am the diamond glint in the snow.
I am the sunlight on the ripened grain.
I am the autumn's gentle rain.

When you awaken in the morning hush,
I am the swift uplifting rush.
Of quiet birds in circled flight.
I am the soft stars
that shine in the night.
Do not stand at my grave and cry.
I am not there.
I did not die.

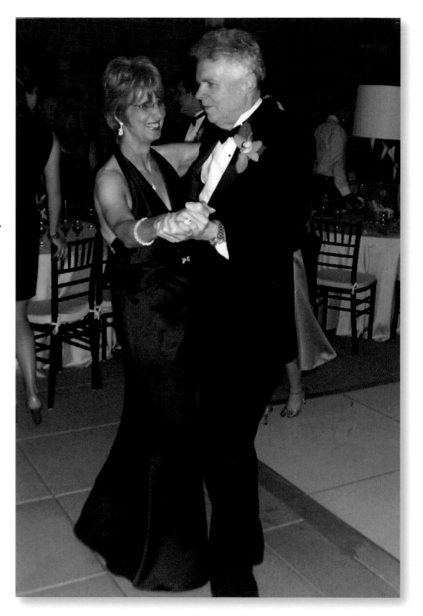

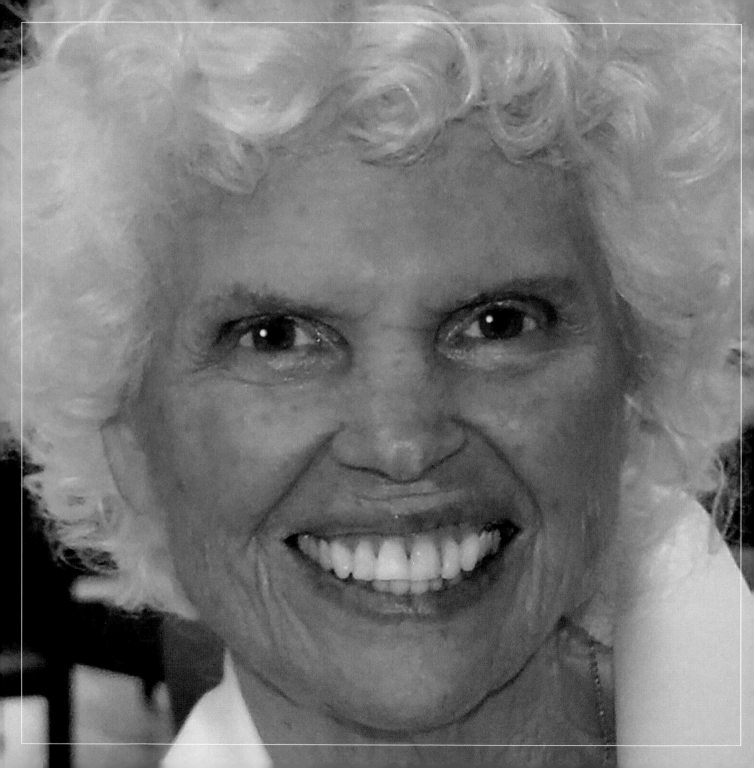

PURPOSE
A Life Still Worth Living

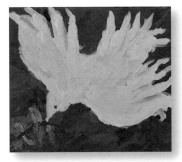

She has always been the type of person who fills up a room. Her beauty—with her striking, curly white hair, bright blue eyes and magnetic smile—are more than enough to attract attention. But it's her inner beauty that radiates as she interacts with others, always looking for ways to shower attention on them. She has a way of making people feel better about themselves in her presence.

So, it wasn't completely surprising when Betty Milner confided to her daughter, Darla, in the car after leaving Amazing Place one day, "I'm so excited! I know why I'm here. God wants me to bring joy to these people. It is my ministry." Even in her dementia, her generous spirit gave her more reason to live.

Once upon a time, Betty had been leader of the "Pirate Belles" drill team, homecoming queen in college, lead singer in the Sweet Adeline's quartet and soloist at her Baptist church. Music always brought her joy. She raised her two young daughters as a single mother after her divorce, working full time in banking to support them. While Darla said they didn't have much growing up, her mom would be the one to lend money to friends. Betty eventually married the love of her life, Sid, who had three children—a son and two daughters and the blended family ended up living an unconventional, but joyful life.

Selling everything they owned in Houston, except for their clothes and two cars, they headed on an adventure, driving through Mexico to land at an isolated, three-mile-long island off the coast of Belize. There, they rented a cottage that looked out on the ocean, bought a boat—aptly named "Benevolence"—and ran a scuba resort. It was primitive living, to say the least. No plumbing, one generator that shut down periodically each day and supplies that arrived once a week by boat. Darla and her siblings attended the one school on the island. They all learned to appreciate the simpler things in life as they fished for lobsters, ate native coconuts and plantains and used palm fronds for privacy.

COMMUNICATING WITH SOMEONE WITH DEMENTIA

Make a connection. A smile and an honest compliment will go miles.

Discuss older milestone memories. Inquire about their first job, first kiss, favorite trip.

Ask about feelings, not facts. "Did you enjoy lunch today?" "Don't you love days like this?" Questions like these have no wrong answers, but asking, "What did you do today?" is very difficult for someone with short-term memory loss to answer.

When you are asked, "Have I told you about..." for the second or third time, reply "Tell me about it." Like all of us, people with dementia want to share and connect; and that's what's important, even if some of the facts aren't quite correct.

If they are stuck on a word or story and keep repeating it, change the environment. Their senses may be picking up the same cues and the repetition will continue. Invite them to another activity or a different room, or play some music they like.

Simplify your questions. As time passes, giving fewer options may be necessary. For example when ordering a meal, instead of asking "What would you like?" ask "Would you like the beef or the chicken?"

Use and ask for non-verbal cues. Sometimes people with dementia can describe what they want better by acting it out.

Eventually returning to Houston, Darla admits, "We definitely had a new perspective on the world. A one-bedroom apartment is a luxury. My mother showed us that life is simple, *we* just make it harder."

No matter where they lived, Darla says that people were always drawn to her mother. "It was like she was always sunshine. She has the ability to see the beauty in everything and has always looked at life as not just half-full, but overflowing."

Thirty years later, Betty, then a widow, was living in a retirement home in Houston near her two daughters. Darla noticed she was losing weight, getting lost and not paying her bills. A self-described clean freak and always one to be put together, she was wearing her clothes inside out. Even then, when she would enter the dining room, she would put a positive spin on it and unapologetically proclaim, "I know it's not right, but here I am!"

Dementia hadn't been on their radars. Darla said, "She'd never been sick or taken a pill," A neurologist confirmed the diagnosis, and Darla and her husband moved in with Betty.

In spite of her mother's vibrant spirit, caregiving was much harder than Darla expected. She was drained with the twenty-four-hour-a-day cycle of care and the emotional toll of watching her mom become more and more like a child. She ended up at a caregiver conference and broke down at a booth for Amazing Place. "It turned out be a blessing for both Mom and me."

In a support group there, Darla learned tools to help her deal with the stress. She found she wasn't alone. "I learned that most caregivers get sicker than their loved ones." Betty, too, found, her place at Amazing Place, where she could shine. In spite of the disease that was stealing her mind, she maintained her indomitable spirit and continued to find ways to fill people up: "Oh, you look so pretty today." "I just love your smile." "That color looks beautiful on you."

> "My mother finds beauty in things that are hard."

Whether she was talking to staff or participants, those on the receiving end of her generous compliments couldn't help but smile back. She was there to help someone who was unsteady out of a chair. She was always looking to lead someone to the next program, holding that person's hands. She was an unofficial

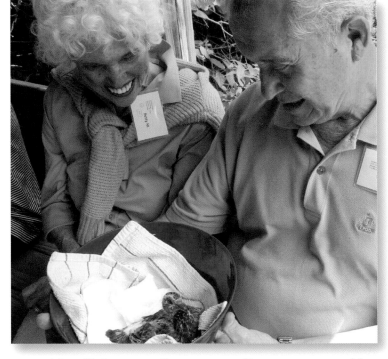

"ambassador," the one who would make new participants feel comfortable. When she missed a day, people noticed. Even when someone said something unkind to her, she would dismiss it and just try that much harder to be nice to them. While people described her as having "Betty Grable" looks, what really drew them to her was her irresistible spirit.

"In her own way, even with her diminishing mind, she continues to be a messenger—someone who sees you as God sees you," says Darla. "She overcomes her own pain by bringing joy to others and at the same time, filling herself up. She finds beauty in things that are hard."

Her life is a reminder that even when you face adversity, you can still share your spirit with the world. And, that in doing so, even with as little as a smile or a compliment, you are able to add joy to another person's life while adding meaning to your own.

FAITH
An Anchor for Life

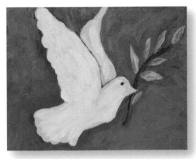

While she suffers from both Parkinson's and Alzheimer's disease, and cannot recall what she just said, or did, Dawn Harrison can share bible verses from memory. She has very limited mobility, and needs assistance to do everything from getting dressed to bathing, but she has an incredible security that she is loved by God. Many people struggle to have an abiding faith when faced with an overwhelming crisis, but Dawn is an inspiring example of maintaining her faith, in spite of an extraordinarily challenging life.

Raised in Jamaica, her steadfast faith began early as her mother and grandmother brought her up in a faith-filled household where church was mandatory. Even today, Dawn says she always trusted God, believing in Him and in what she learned at church. She recalls once when she was a little girl and didn't want to go to church, she told her mother that she was sick. Her mother, sensing she was making up an excuse, replied, "Dawn, you just need to go on to church, and they will pray for you to get well."

At twenty-six, she married and had three daughters, Marlene, Michelle and Monique. Dawn did her best to keep a happy atmosphere in her home, preparing fresh Jamaican food for her family, finding humor in things and making sure that her darling girls were always well-dressed, especially for Sunday church.

In 1980, Dawn realized she needed to make a change to provide a better life for her and her daughters. In one of the hardest decisions of her life, she left Jamaica by herself and came to the US, where she ended up working two jobs, at Walgreen's and Houston Methodist Hospital, while also attending Houston Community College to get her nursing prerequisites. She sent money back to her family and big boxes of clothes, shoes and non-perishable groceries—all with the hope of one day bringing her children to Texas.

During this difficult time away from her children, her belief that God was with her and her children never faltered. Her anchor was her faith from childhood and whenever she felt things would never get better, she would remember the verse from Deuteronomy 31:8 *"The Lord himself goes before you and will be with you, He will never leave you nor forsake you. Do not be afraid; do not be discouraged."* She says she always trusted that "God would never forget us: He would forgive us, and He is good."

Her children eventually moved to Texas and made lives for themselves while Dawn worked as a secretary at Houston Methodist Hospital. In 2008, one of the doctors at Houston Methodist noticed Dawn was having tremors. Diagnosed with Parkinson's disease, she moved in with her daughter Marlene and continued to work. When her tremors progressed, she ended up having a DBS (deep brain stimulation) procedure in 2012, during which bleeding in the blood vessels in the frontal lobe impaired her short-term memory. While she still yearned to work, she was unable to continue due to her memory loss.

Marlene says that in all the years her mother had worked, she had never taken a vacation. Now, suddenly, she was at home all the time, and she missed having a purpose. Dawn would listen to the Christian radio station KSBJ during the day, watch Joyce Meyer's television ministry every morning, read her prayer book and go to church each Sunday.

Gradually, over the next year, Dawn started repeating things and displaying symptoms that resulted in a diagnosis of Alzheimer's disease. Her daughters realized their mother would benefit from a day center for those with dementia and Amazing Place became Dawn's home away from home during the week. It was there that she developed a new purpose— attending bible study faithfully each day, where a leader shares a lesson, followed by hymns and prayer requests.

WHY A DEMENTIA DAY PROGRAM?

Research continues to support the many benefits of a day program for those with dementia and their caregivers. A good day program should provide:

- Social stimulation

- Cognitive stimulation

- Physical stimulation with daily exercise

- Spiritual stimulation–bible study

- Brain healthy nutrition

- Daily health care monitoring with on-site registered nurse

- Respite, support and decreased stress for caregivers

- Cost effectiveness in comparison to in-home care

After lunch at Amazing Place, Dawn slowly makes her way to the chapel with a walker, determined to be on time. It's not unusual for her to quote a bible verse, whisper soft, while she takes each deliberate step: *"Trust in the Lord with all your heart and lean not unto your own understanding. In all your ways acknowledge Him and He will make your paths straight."* Her face is particularly radiant when she shares bible verses from memory, demonstrating that even Alzheimer's cannot remove these verses from her heart and mind. When she enters the chapel, Dawn lovingly greets everyone as she struggles to get seated in one of the chairs around a big table. She graciously thanks her fellow participants who offer her assistance to get seated.

During the bible study, Dawn recites lengthy scriptures, quietly sings hymns and exchanges encouraging and uplifting words with her friends. She is not alone, as each person around the table, in spite of their dementia, reflects an unwavering assurance about their faith and support for each other. They all are living proof that God has a special love for those who appear weak in the eyes of the world, and they serve as powerful conduits of grace to one another.

Each person, in spite of their dementia, reflects an unwavering assurance about their faith.

One particular day, another participant in the bible study group seemed to be particularly fearful and inconsolable. Dawn sensed her friend's anxiety, and painstakingly rose, holding on to the table for support. Looking at her friend with a steady gaze, she began quoting from Psalm 121: *I lift up my eyes to the hills—where does my help come from? My help comes from the Lord, the Maker of heaven and earth.* Sharing word-for-word the majority of the psalm, she then said to everyone "I love you…I need to go now," leaving earlier than usual to go to an appointment. She leaned on her walker and slowly made her way down the hall, while everyone responded, "We love you, too!"

Today, it's her daughters' turn to care for their mother, making sure she is beautifully attired, able to attend Amazing Place and see her grandchildren. While Dawn may forget things in the short term, she is quick to say to each of her daughters, "I love you…I love you *more*!"

One of the verses Dawn loves to quote, Psalm 91:1-2, sums up her rock-solid faith: *He who dwells in the shelter of the Most High will rest in the shadow of the Almighty. I will say of the Lord, "He is my refuge and my fortress, my God in whom I trust."* Fortunately for Dawn, her Parkinson's and Alzheimer's have allowed her to retain her long-term memories. She remembers fondly her childhood days in Jamaica and her career at Methodist. But what is most moving is how her trust in God continues to anchor her. Parkinson's and Alzheimer's disease will never take it away.

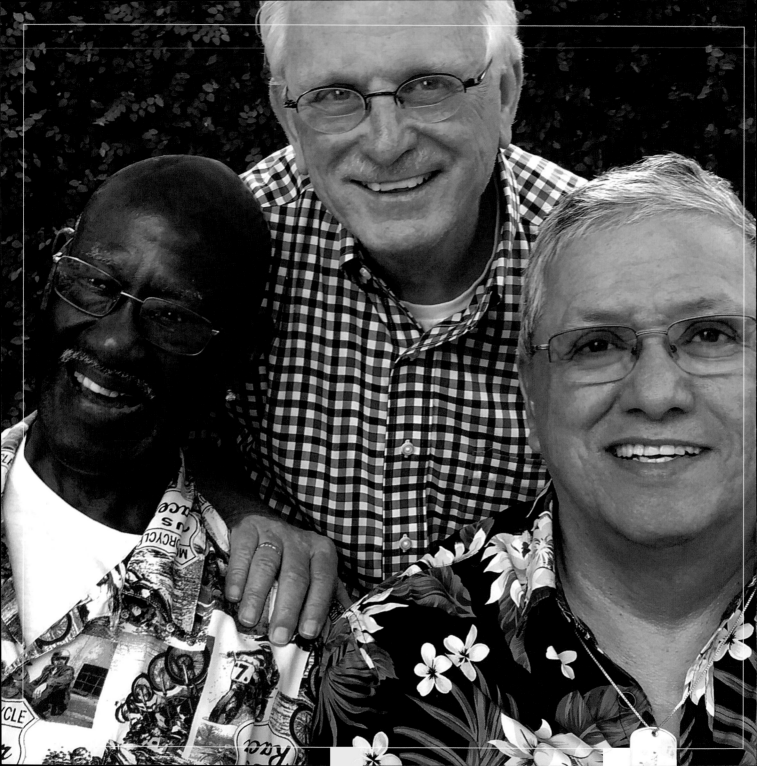

CONNECTIONS

When Labels Vanish

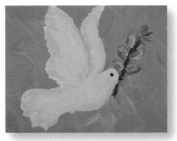

They came from three very different backgrounds, led three very different lives, yet late in life, they found a common bond. One friend is a former company executive, a triathlete and father to two adopted Vietnamese girls who are now teenagers. Another is a retired electronic component repairman with a passion for music, who played keyboard, recorded albums and toured with a number of Tejano bands. And the third is a Korean War veteran, barber and truck driver with a fondness for all things Creole, from crawfish to Zydeco music. Each man found his way to Amazing Place after being diagnosed with dementia. There, they developed a friendship that, like any true friendship, includes trust, safety and plain old fun.

JERRY

Jerry Bates readily admits he had a rough childhood with two alcoholic parents. But he believes it's what drove him to need to control his life and helped him accomplish so much in his career. A cheerleader in college, it was there that he determined to turn his life around and be successful. He graduated with a degree in business and moved quickly up the corporate ladder to eventually become a chief operating officer at Arthur J. Gallagher & Co., a Fortune 500 firm.

That intense focus carried over to his personal life, where he completed fourteen marathons after recovering from testicular cancer in his thirties. He met his match, Betsy, at a church dance, where she says she learned, "He loved to dance and was crazy like me!" A lawyer and accountant and equally passionate, she became his second wife, and she encouraged him to join her in triathlons.

Relatively late in life—Betsy was forty-seven and Jerry was fifty-eight—they adopted twin girls, Brittany and Brianna, from Vietnam. After three grueling trips back and forth to Vietnam, they finally brought the girls home when they were eighteen months old.

Betsy says Jerry never met a stranger and has always been the life of the party. He is an extremely loyal friend and still attends Texans football games with his close friend of forty-five years, Mike Turner.

At an annual physical, Jerry's astute internist detected some signs of memory issues when he said he was having trouble with numbers, his previous strong suit. A neurologist confirmed the unexpected diagnosis of Alzheimer's, which Jerry acknowledges has changed the course of their lives. He admits, "It has been the ultimate test in letting go." Betsy, a manager of International Tax at Deloitte, now juggles her demanding career with managing the finances and household matters, as well as parenting their twins, now teens. She admits it's been a big adjustment to take on all the decisions Jerry once made.

Knowing how social Jerry was, she found Amazing Place for him to attend while she worked. He says he "loves it here" and Betsy adds that he misses it on the weekends. He also divulges, "It's helpful to be able to talk candidly with others who are facing similar challenges." His gregariousness is evident, and you can often hear him engaging with friends, dancing or sharing a hearty laugh.

ALFRED

It turns out Jerry's first day was also the same day Alfred Luna started at Amazing Place, and perhaps that initial introduction is what started their bond. Music has always been Alfred's lifeline. In middle school, he started playing keyboard with a Tejano band, Sunny and the Sunliners. Their music took off; they had a top hit, "Talk to Me," and they started playing bigger and bigger venues, including opening for Franke Valle and the Four Seasons at the Houston Coliseum. Alfred left high school to tour around the country with the group, but he soon found he was not often allowed into many of the clubs because of his age.

"We have each other's back."

Returning to Houston to finish high school and graduate from community college, he was soon drafted into the Army during the height of the Vietnam War. After being injured during basic training, he stayed at Camp Pendleton, where many of his Army buddies couldn't believe he was on the radio.

Returning home in 1973 after his military stint, he returned to his passion and joined the band Rocky Gil & the Bishops. He wrote and recorded the title song on their album, "Soul Party" as well as "After Party" and "It's Not the End." Alfred married his high school sweetheart, and they had three children. To allow him flexibility for his music gigs and the ability to support his family, he worked repairing electronic components in vending machines for many years. He continued to play with many Tejano bands including The Saints and Sinners Band up until a few years ago.

In 2004, divorced, he was at a friend's house where he ran into the sister of his former middle school flame. Forty-two years after their initial friendship, Alfred and Dolores connected. She, also divorced, claims she had no intention of marrying again. "But he started calling every day," she says, "and I couldn't get him off my back." At a church fundraiser six months later, Alfred asked her to marry him.

Just two years later, Dolores started noticing some memory and behavior changes in Alfred. He had a hard time with money, he jerked a lot while he slept, and he kept losing things. Since then, three different neurologists have given him three different diagnoses: Lewy body dementia, frontotemporal dementia and Alzheimer's disease. More recently, Dolores has noticed his anxiety has increased and his memory has worsened, in spite of the medications he's been taking.

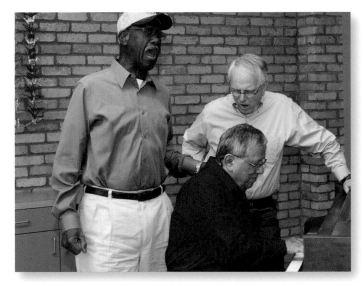

Like Betsy, Dolores found Amazing Place as a place for her husband to attend while she works full time—as an office manager at a dental office. Dolores says if Alfred is home, all he does is watch TV, and he gets very upset when he can't go to Amazing Place. Characteristic of those who have Alzheimer's, he has lost his concept of day and time, which can cause problems with expectations "Last Easter Sunday," Dolores says, "Alfred was dressed and ready to go at six am to Amazing Place and was upset to learn he couldn't go."

She accepts the reality of his illness, and says that "God put us together for a reason: so I could take care of him." Alfred has not lost his ability to play piano, although he can no longer read music. The deep, long-term memories of many songs have stayed with him, and he continues to play for family and friends in their studio at their home. When he sits down at the piano at Amazing Place, participants and staff also get the benefit of his remarkable talent.

FOSTER
The third member of this trio of friends, Blume "Foster" Foster, will quickly tell you he's from Hearne, Texas, then spell, "H-E-A-R-N-E" and ask if you know where it is. Foster fought in the Korean War and is fluent in Korean in addition to Cajun. He and his wife adopted a daughter, Zora.

A PRESCRIPTION FOR BRAIN HEALTHY LIVING: WHAT'S GOOD FOR YOUR HEART AND SOUL IS ALSO GOOD FOR YOUR BRAIN

Regular physical activity increases blood and oxygen flow to the brain. Ideally, 150 minutes of moderate-intensity exercise per week is recommended by the American Heart Association.

Reduce cardiovascular risks, for example, diabetes, obesity, smoking and hypertension, which can impact cognitive health.

Eat a healthy diet emphasizing whole grains, fruits and vegetables, fish and shellfish, nuts, olive oil and other healthy fats; and reducing saturated fats and red meat.

Continue to learn and keep your mind engaged.

Maintain social connections.

Find effective ways to manage stress.

Engage in a spiritual practice that can help you cope with illness, depression and anxiety.

When she was six, they divorced, and Zora grew up with her mother who was a beautician. Foster worked first as a barber and then as an eighteen-wheeler driver. In addition to his passion for Creole food, Zora says he has always loved music and dancing. It wasn't unusual for him to walk around with headphones on, or go on stage at a club and start singing the blues. There was always music around their house—guitars and organs. Foster's other passions, as he will tell you, are the Green Bay Packers and LA Dodgers, and he is frequently seen wearing a Packers shirt or a Dodgers hat.

A few years ago, Zora was working in real estate in Dallas and divorced with a son in college, when she received a call from the VA doctors that her father needed someone to take care of him. Her mother had died, and she was all the family he had. While he had recovered from both prostate and stomach cancers, he was now exhibiting signs of Alzheimer's disease—forgetting and losing things—and the doctors determined it was no longer safe for him to live alone.

Zora had to move to Houston, selling her house and finding a new job. She admits the difficulty of the situation and says it "has pretty much overtaken my life." She adds, "We both had an adjustment. He didn't like the fact that, as his daughter, I was taking control." But she says her father has slowly realized he can no longer be in total control of his life. The VA recommended Amazing Place as a support for both Zora and Foster and, like Jerry and Alfred, he says he wants to go there every day.

THE TRIO

Each day, at lunch at Amazing Place, you'll find these three men sitting together. Sometimes they're hooting and hollering; other times, talking about the latest ball game. After lunch, it's not surprising to find Alfred playing the piano, while Foster sings a Zydeco song and Jerry dances along. One of the staff members at Amazing Place has dubbed them "The Three Amigos."

Talking to each of them about the others is when you really understand their bond. Jerry says, "Alfred is a best friend, caring, concerned about me. We have each other's back. I help him out when he gets lost (walking around at Amazing Place) and he does the same for me...And Foster, well, he's always funny and entertaining...you never know what he's going to come out with."

Alfred adds, "I like how I can talk about the way I feel and talk freely and don't feel like anyone is judging me. It's like we're related to one another."

Finally Foster chimes in, saying, "I like that they treat me like a brother. Jerry and I both like crawfish. Jerry likes to tease me, and we all like music."

In this safe, nurturing environment where diverse individuals have lost certain faculties, facades and labels disappear. Friendships like that of Jerry, Alfred and Foster can flourish. When what is unimportant in life is stripped away, it is easy to see that we are all equal and valuable in the eyes of God.

REMEMBER THIS

The families who have shared their stories here are just a very few of the courageous individuals who have been part of Amazing Place for the last twenty years. It is easy to recite facts and figures and speak of how many people are served by a mission such as this, but that information will never tell the whole story.

It is our hope that by learning more about some of the unique men and women who have found community and caring here in a time of transition and uncertainty, you have a better understanding not only of dementia, but also of the grace we witness every day. Yes, a diagnosis of dementia is frightening, and the demands it places on families can be overwhelming. But the participants at Amazing Place show us, over and over again, that while dementia may change some of their memory, thinking and behavior, it does not take away their need for dignity and for finding meaning and purpose each day. And, it cannot destroy what is most important: faith, hope and love.

While we do not have a cure for dementia, these families show us that we need not fear it. Each of them mourns the loss of the individual they have known, but they have embraced the loving soul who remains. Their stories reveal that dementia is not the destruction of what is most important, but it is a paring back to what is most essential. It can bring walls down and allow us to connect in ways we may never have dreamed possible. And, these stories share lessons for all of us about how to live life with courage, gratitude and acceptance.

If you or a family member has been diagnosed with dementia, you do not walk alone. There are resources, support and companions for this part of the journey. Your local Alzheimer's Association chapter is a great place to start. At Amazing Place, our mission is to provide a safe place to land and a place of hope for those in the Houston area. We trust that as the population ages and more families deal with dementia, there will be more "amazing places" for support.

In the end, whether we have dementia or have our mind fully intact, it is worth remembering that what really matters is that faith, hope and love can anchor us through life. The greatest of these is love; and, even in the face of dementia, love never fails.

SPECIAL THANKS TO ...

The twelve individuals and families featured in this book whose willingness and courage to be vulnerable and share their personal stories will have a profound impact on the perception of dementia.

Tracey Brown, Amazing Place Executive Director,
who was instrumental in conceiving and supporting this project from the beginning.

Sharon Tooley,
for the donation of her beautiful concept design.

Photographer Cindy Crofford and Digital Artist Diane Murphy
who donated their extraordinary talents in photography.
(Photos on pages 20, 38, 44, 58, 65, 72).

Susan Giles, Amazing Place Community and Church Liaison,
who was kind and thorough in interviewing,
researching and drafting
Dawn Harrison's story about Faith.

Lauren Gow and Fiona Bills of Bright Sky Press for
their invaluable help in steering the process of creating a book.

Finally, Lucy Chambers of Bright Sky Press,
who provided expert and sensitive direction and input
for this project from the very beginning of concept
development through the final draft.

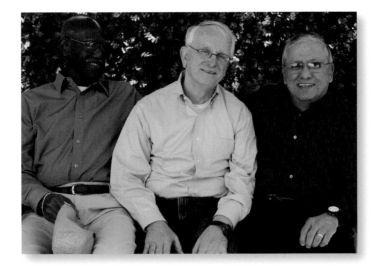

REMEMBER...
THEY STILL HAVE
MUCH TO CONTRIBUTE
AND
MUCH TO TEACH US.

AMAZING PLACE
20TH ANNIVERSARY

PROVIDING FELLOWSHIP,
MEMORY CARE
AND WELLNESS
FOR ADULTS
WITH MILD TO
MODERATE DEMENTIA
AND SUPPORT
TO THEIR FAMILIES
AND THE COMMUNITY
SINCE 1996.

20 YEARS
OF
REMEMBERING
WHAT MATTERS

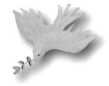